The Hands That Feed Me

Introducing the
SOFT AIM Approach
for Recovery from Compulsive Eating

Annette McLean
LCPC, CEDS

outskirts
press

"I usually don't like self-help books, even though I have been drawn to many. I begin them full of hope, yet time and again they falter soon after the introduction or first chapter, and I lose interest. But Ms. McLean's "been there, done that" style, combines scientific data and research, a clinical approach from her years of therapeutic counseling, and a healthy dose of healing spirituality and mindfulness to make this book a winner! I had more than one AHA moment and even several WOW moments, but most importantly I feel this book will guide readers to turn that corner and realize they are ready to use her tools to guide them in their own recovery. Her SOFT AIM technique, borne from equal parts study, counseling, and personal recovery, will let readers lean into their sacred journey."

Patty H.

Annette McLean's *The Hands That Feeds Me* is an elegant symphony of clinical knowledge, the skills necessary to recover from binge eating, with a chorus of personal understanding thrown in. Annette's experience with her own food issues, combined with her decades of professional experience are reflected in the development of the SOFT AIM approach. As a therapist, I have used the SOFT AIM approach with my clients who struggle with binge eating and have found it to be extremely helpful. This is a must-read for anyone who struggles with binge eating or any professional who treats them.

Julie Barthels, LCSW, ACS

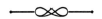

THE HANDS THAT FEED ME maps out a brilliant path toward healing. The SOFT AIM approach is straightforward and clear, deep and wise. Annette McLean combines story and structure with a conversational tone that makes you feel like she's right there with you. Solid and timely science combined with a depth of soul and spiritual inquiry makes this a unique recovery process. SOFT AIM will invigorate your recovery and bring your life to a whole new level of healing, one step at a time, gently and powerfully.

Dina L.

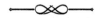

Dedication
To my clients, the bravest people I know

Table of Contents

CHAPTER 1

Welcome to the Wild Ride

And I said to my body softly, "I want to be your friend." It took a long breath. And replied, "I have been waiting my whole life for this."

-Nayyirah Waheed

My Twisted Path to Recovery

The roots of my own eating disorder began when I was very young. I was an anxious child and a ridiculously picky eater. By age six I was unhealthy and underweight. After a health scare and a visit to Mayo Clinic, my well-meaning parents were determined to "fatten me up." Dinner time became a battle. I also learned that eating brought lavish praise and comments of what a "good girl" I was. Added to this was my Sicilian heritage and the cultural emphasis on "Mangia, mangia, mangia!" which translates to "Eat, eat, eat!" The seeds were well planted. Food was love, and love was food.

But it was around the time of my parents' divorce and my adolescence that my eating disorder really began. I even remember the moment that body confidence turned into body dissatisfaction. We were on a family vacation at a rustic cabin on a lake. I was excited that I had been allowed to bring my best friend, Suzy. That first morning, we woke bright and early and put on our bikinis. I loved that swimsuit. It was black cotton with little orange flowers and bright green leaves. I remember the day well. It was a gorgeous summer morning. We were headed to the dock to take out the clumsy rowboat. We planned on sunning ourselves all day. We packed snacks and drinks and then realizing we had not had breakfast, we decided to make banana splits. This was a vacation after all. Giggling we made our decadent dessert breakfasts. We even put cherries and whip cream on top. As we walked barefoot through the June grass, bikini clad with sundaes in hand, my uncle and his friend stopped their conversation to turn and stare. "You better be careful," my uncle admonished. "You are starting to get fat."

Not that it matters, but I was far from fat. Perhaps my budding sexuality made him uncomfortable? I will never know. But if I am to name the moment that my own eating disorder began, this was it. Two weeks later, another male relative made a similar comment. That sealed it. The bikini was packed away forever. The quest for thinness was born. My own alternate reality was created. Deprivation became my religion and from the restriction came the binging.

My restrictions were creative: the apple a day diet, the water only fasts, the 500 calorie diets, the cabbage soup diet, and the chew food up and spit it out diet. Then of course came the binges. From my hunger grew the compulsion to stuff myself with as much food as possible. All efforts to control intake were followed by equally uncontrolled binges. Binges were of a grand and enormous scale. I would routinely go through drive-thrus, eat the food, and then immediately drive through another one to do it again. I had a short stint of binging and purging, and a too long stint of amphetamines. In my early 20's, I was diagnosed with a heart disorder called mitral valve prolapse. I suspect that my eating disorder caused it.

My body image was distorted. I could look in the mirror in the morning with a flatter stomach and on a good day say, "Ok, not bad." Then have a normal lunch a few hours later, look in the same mirror and be sure I had grown three sizes. So deep were my distortions that I was certain that I could literally *feel* my fat cells expanding after eating. I would lament to those around me that I felt fat. Truly, I physically "felt" that sensation all over my body.

Finally, all of the restricting and binging caught up with me. As a result of yo-yo dieting, I started to gain weight in spite of my efforts to eat normally. By now, I was a grown-up and a mom. I tried more conventional and "sensible" diets. Nothing worked for long. I was obsessed with food, my body size, and the scale. Every morning my first thought of the day was "How did I do yesterday?" This, of course, meant, "Did I stick to the diet?" By that time, my behavior was typical of most compulsive eaters. I was a saint by day (under-eating), but because I was tired and starving when I got home from work, I binged my way through the night. This, of course meant that I had broken yet another promise to myself. I felt depressed, ashamed, and hopeless.

Eventually, I realized that it was recovery I needed, not another diet. I was using food and restriction of food to soothe emotional pain and cope with problems.

I read every book on recovery I could find. I combined techniques. Some days I was strictly an intuitive eater, allowing my hunger and satiety to dictate my eating. Then something would happen and I would start to compulsively eat again. Days would turn to weeks. I would then put myself on a meal plan and remove the triggers from the house for a while. I went on like this for a long time. I am not going to give you a play-by-play account of my recovery because we are all different. Suffice to say, my journey of recovery was filled with countless twists and turns.

The Wisdom of Imperfection

As a therapist, telling you such a personal story is a controversial move. We, as counseling professionals, are taught to be very careful about self-disclosure. However, I have come to realize that my recovery affords a needed sense of hope for my clients. Research shows that working with someone who is recovered provides a sense of inspiration for those struggling with disordered eating.[1]

One of the problems I encountered while writing this book is my pronoun usage. I have alternated between being at one with you, the reader, and with being the psychotherapist and eating disorder professional. I ask you, dear reader, not to be confused by this, as the reality is *I am* both the person who has struggled with disordered eating and the professional who, by treating it, has a level of expertise.

Some of you may be new to the path, some seasoned. Either way, my hope is to inspire and assist you. Most importantly, I will provide you with the basic tools of recovery as well as with a coping tool I created called, SOFT AIM.

So, why else do I write this book? Well, I AM a licensed therapist and a certified eating disorder specialist. I have several years of experience treating eating disorders in my private practice. I guess that makes me somewhat qualified. But that is not why I write this book.

One of the greatest gifts of recovery is my increased and now regular contact with my inner guidance system. Indeed, this inner guidance communicates with me whenever I ask and sometimes even when I don't. It provides wisdom, clarity, and always a deeper truth.

Recently, I was on a plane headed for a conference. Trips give me an opportunity to tune into my inner guidance system. I find I reflect and think best when I journal. So, on this trip I was writing about my plans for the coming year. I had pretty much decided that I was going to apply for a Masters in Medicinal Herbalism program. For the past year, I had been taking classes in the uses of herbs. I learned to make tonics and tinctures for coughs and colds and other maladies. I learned about wild plants that are not only edible but also superbly good for us. I felt more grounded and closer to the earth than ever before, and I was excited about my new knowledge. Indeed, I felt "called" to further study the uses of medicinal herbs.

So, there I sat journaling about what I thought was an obvious decision. When I journal, I often write in dialogue form, like a conversation with my intuition. However, instead of affirmations for what I thought was my new found passion, I found myself writing the words: "No, not this year."

"What? But why? How could this be the wrong direction?" I

argued. Then I wrote, plain as day, "You need to write a book about recovery. You can't do both. It's too much. If you really want to, you can do the herbalism program later." I thought, but didn't write, "This is crazy." But I am sure this conversation came from a sense of intuitive knowing. In short, it felt "right."

Following the internal argument came the self-doubt. I wrote, "My recovery has been a long, drawn out, crazy mess." After which came the response: "Who better? You are just right for this in your imperfection." So, that was it. New marching orders. I have learned it is better to listen to my intuition than not. And from that dialogue was born the idea for this book.

Our stories may be similar or very different. That, my friend, is not important. Just know that I understand how deep this struggle goes. I lift up a prayer that the words in this book can help you through the doorway and onto the path of your own recovery.

How to Use this Book

Although I am one who likes to jump around in a self-help book, I am going to suggest that you start at the beginning and work through this book in a linear fashion. The first few chapters provide you with the "bones" or mechanics of recovery. You will need these just to establish some sanity around food as you learn the rest of the recovery skills. The process of recovery begins by becoming conscious of how the disorder manifests in you. This is the beginning of what will become our practice of mindfulness. It is about becoming conscious of the disorder, learning to eat according to physical hunger and then, the often more challenging part, of learning what is enough. Most of the remainder of the book explains the SOFT AIM Approach for recovery. SOFT AIM will be an effective tool in learning to recognize and regulate emotions and thoughts. And most importantly, it will help you develop your inner guidance. The last chapter entitled "Pulling it Together" is about just that; putting the tools together to create your own recovery. Take as long as you need with each chapter. Set a goal and make it realistic to your life and needs. This is important work.

If you set aside the time to read AND do the homework, you will get more out of this book.

Basic Tools

- Buy a journal or download a digital diary online. Have it next to you when you pick up this book. Don't worry that what you write seems nonsensical or "crazy." Write for your own eyes. Write the truth. If you don't write the truth, writing is a waste of time. Dr. James W. Pennebaker, a social psychologist at the University of Texas at Austin, is considered to be the pioneer of writing therapy. His basic paradigm for expressive writing remains widely used today. He advises you to write without concern for grammar, sentence structure or spelling. Says Pennebaker: "When people are given the opportunity to write about emotional upheavals, they often experience improved health. They go to the doctor less. They even have changes in immune function."[2]

- Don't merely read this book. Write your homework assignments. Journal your reactions, thoughts, anything that interests you or doesn't interest you. Joan Didion once said: "I don't know what I think until I write about it." You will get greater benefits from this book if you stop to do the assignments and exercises as you go. Often, I have clients tell me that they have not written their homework but "know it in their head." Writing it does and will make a difference. Taking thoughts out of your head and putting them on paper is often necessary for clarity.

- Find the right support. If you do not already have a therapist and it is at all possible to get one, do so. The same is true for a dietician. For both, try to find someone versed in eating disorders and who has an understanding of cognitive behavioral therapy. Sometimes, we have deeper issues and traumas that need healing if we are going to be able to fully recover. The help of a therapist is worth the time, effort and money. The assistance of a support group, too, can be a wonderful adjunct to your recovery. Check in your area to see if anything like this is available. Family and friends can be fantastic additions to your support team as well. Just know they may need to be educated in this approach to be of real help.

- This is NOT the time to embark on a new diet. Diets take a great deal of energy. If you focus your energy on trying to lose weight right now, you will not be able to focus on recovery. Sometimes we do naturally lose weight as an outcome of no longer binging, but think of it as a possible side effect, not the goal. At least not now. You need to get off this "crazy train" of binging followed by dieting to allow your body to stabilize at a weight. If you diet now, you will likely repeat the same cycle. You need to trust this process.

Journal Assignment

1. What is your story? Did your childhood play into your disordered eating? How? What has been the nature of your "wild ride" with food and weight? Write about it. Alternatively, find a trusted person to talk with about it.

2. Do you believe that you can recover from disordered eating? Do you really want to?

CHAPTER **2**

Waking Up

The wound is the place where the light enters you.

-Rumi

This chapter is about making the unconscious, conscious. It is about putting a long, lovely crack into the ceiling of that stone cave that is compulsive eating. Once the crack forms, allowing the light to shine through, there is no turning back. You may forget a thousand times, but you will always return to that place where the light enters, and nothing will ever be quite the same. This consciousness is where re-covery begins.

I believe that one of the reasons why a change of this magnitude is so difficult is because many of our thoughts and behaviors are be-ing run automatically by our subconscious. Neuroscientists have dis-covered that almost 80% of the neural instructions for our behavior are hard wired into our implicit memory.[1] This means they run on auto-pilot. For example, if you were in a car accident at 7 years old, you will likely remember the event. You can consciously process this memory. This is an example of explicit memory. If however, you were in a car accident at 7 months, you have no context to consciously re-member or understand the event. Your body, however, will remember and respond automatically. You may wonder why you fear riding in cars in spite of evidence that you are safe. We can blame "implicit

8

memory" for many of our dysfunctional behaviors.

Even when we are older and can remember events, we may forget them. They will however, still be stored as implicit memory. These implicit memories will affect our choices and behaviors in ways we often do not understand. Add to this the fact that our coping style is firmly encoded in our neural network by 18 months.[2] Our coping style is chosen *for* us, not by us. We literally default and act in milliseconds to any perceived threat.

To ensure our survival, we also have what scientists have termed "negativity bias".[3] Our ancestors knew they were better off jumping away from a stick that looked like a snake than examining it and later deciding what to do. They were the ones who were anxious about that last piece of fruit on the apple tree. Those that decided to nap and worry later about food were likely to starve. That we have this bias is a "given." But the strength is determined during our first year and a half of life by how well our caregivers provided safety and comfort. The stronger the negativity bias, the more difficulty we have coping, and the more likely we are to use food to self-soothe.

The good news is that evolution also gave us a capacity for resilience. The not so good news is that how well that innate capacity develops and matures depends once again, on our learned patterns of responding to situations. Some of us did not have the best examples. Some of us had traumas that overwhelmed our resources or abilities to cope.

Thankfully neuroscientists have also discovered a concept called neuroplasticity.[4] This term refers to our ability to rewire and rebuild brain structures. This means we no longer have to be victims of our limited coping strategies. We can learn to be more resilient. We can learn to cope without food.

This book will introduce you to a coping tool I have created called SOFT AIM. You will learn specific strategies through SOFT AIM that will help you change the neural pathways in your brain connected to your disordered eating and, thus, become more resilient. SOFT AIM is both a descriptor and an acronym. It is a "descriptor" because aiming softly is how you will approach this journey. It is an acronym because each letter stands for a skill you will learn to become more resilient. I am confident that it will be a useful tool for your recovery. SOFT AIM is based on everything I have learned about eating disorders and healing. The specifics of this approach will be outlined and explained as we go along. For now, however, let's talk more about this thing called recovery.

I used to call it a path. But recovery as a path denotes steps, and this may lead you into thinking that this process is linear. Let me be clear. Recovery from compulsive eating is anything but linear. I also used to liken it to climbing Mount Everest in a blizzard. Two steps forward, one step back, and you cannot even see the destination you are aspiring towards. But now I realize that if indeed this is Mount Everest, all that happens at the top is that now you need to jump. Jenni Schaefer in her book, *Goodbye Ed, Hello Me*, says that the free fall is that leap of faith that one must take for full recovery; it is that point where you are going to trust the process without stipulations.[5]

So, what else is recovery? For one, it is individualized. Just as no two individuals are the same, no two recoveries will be exactly alike. What works for you may not work for the next person, and vice versa. If you are looking for a cookie cutter, one size fits all recovery book, you will not find it within these pages.

If you are looking for something you can execute in short order perfection, you will be disappointed as well. Recovery is imperfect. If it were a color, it would be gray. We usually want black or white answers to things, but black and white thinking is part of the problem. Our culture, which is diet and weight obsessed, promotes this type of all or nothing thinking. Diets say we are either "on" or "off", and if we "blew it", hell, we might as well have a party until tomorrow or Monday or New Year's Day or January 2nd.

Think about it. Food is not like an addiction to alcohol or drugs where complete abstinence is desirable or even possible. Food will forever be ambiguous. Was this too much or too little? Was I hungry enough? We may have trigger foods that incite a binge, caused by emotional cues or years of deprivation rather than a true chemical addiction to food. Disordered eating is more of a process addiction. We are addicted to the process of binging, not the food itself. That said, we are now learning that food manufacturers have managed to create certain foods that do have an addictive quality to them. Many highly processed foods can cause excess hunger and stimulate brain regions involved in reward and cravings.[6] This is yet another reason recovery from compulsive eating is so complicated.

Recovery is making peace with food and our body. That is, I know, a tall order. For years we have not trusted ourselves or our appetites. Until we take a break from the calorie counter and diet book, we will never fully recover. Until we find compassion for ourselves, we will stay stuck in this hamster wheel. We cannot hate ourselves into recovery. And don't be fooled into thinking you can just hate your stomach or your thighs but not yourself. The hatred you feel for your body eventually becomes hatred for your entire self.

Recovery is not primarily about losing weight. There may be a time for that, but it is not now. It cannot be the main goal. If it is, recovery just turns into the new diet. And as we all know, diets have not worked. How often have you and the people you know lost and regained all of the lost weight plus some? I do not believe for a minute that *we* fail on all of those diets. I DO however believe that all those diets fail us. They do not address the correct set of problems. They wrongly assume overeaters simply lack willpower. If it were only that simple. It is very important for you to understand that you are not in this situation because you are a moral failure. You have developed maladaptive patterns with food and weight for complex reasons. Perhaps it was the only way you knew how to care for yourself. Maybe it is the way you calm yourself. As the poet Maya Angelou wrote: "When you know better, you do better."

Historically, we have put overeaters in a different category than those with anorexia nervosa or bulimia nervosa. If you are anorexic or bulimic, the medical and behavioral health community has recognized that emotional factors must be addressed as well as medical issues.

It is only recently, however, that the health community has come to understand this is also true of overeaters. Why it has taken so long is a discourse best left for another book. It is frustrating to say the least.

Recovery is a process, not an event. This is another way of saying that it may take a long time. I say this not to dishearten, but rather to validate you. Once again, it is important to realize that you are not in this situation because you are undisciplined. That is not the case at all. There is a saying in the recovery movement something to the effect of, "Your worst day in recovery is better than your best day as an addict." I could not agree more. Recovery from compulsive eating is often fraught with starts and stops. Yes, more imperfection. That's okay. The good news is you can recover if you keep working at it, one eating experience at a time.

Recovery from disordered eating takes courage. For most of us, it will be the bravest thing we ever do. Why? For one thing, it requires being completely honest with ourselves. It requires facing every emotion and facing every situation that we have done our damnedest to avoid through disordered eating.

Binges, especially, are something we need to make conscious. This, too, is difficult since mindlessness is the nature of the binge. We are not tasting when binging, not really. We are not grateful, nor are we noticing the subtle flavors, the aromas, or the textures. We are not truly present for the event. Binges are mechanical. At times they are nearly maniacal. Pity the friend or family member that interrupts the binge in progress.

You must make everything about your disordered eating conscious as well. How do you eat? Is it fast or slow? Where do you eat? Is it in the car or is it in secret? Do you allow yourself to be in full view of others? When do you eat? Most overeaters are saints (aka *restrictors* in the diet world) by day and let loose in the evenings. What are your patterns? What are the things that trigger your overeating? Do not worry if you do not know the answer to this last question. Unearthing this is much of what this book is about.

You also must wake up to your self-talk. What happens if your jeans are tight? What happens when you step on the scale? What is your commentary when you look into a mirror or catch your reflection in a shop window? What thoughts are running through your mind about you every day?

I do an exercise in my therapy groups that focuses on self-talk. I ask the women to write on a sheet of paper one of the worst things they say about themselves. I ask them to write in second person with a "you" as opposed to an "I". They laugh as they come up with a horrid thing they say. They write, for example, "You are a disgusting fat blob," and "Your stomach is as large as your butt." The mood is light while they are trying to outdo each other in their wicked statements. Then I say, "Okay, now turn to the person to your right, put her name at the beginning of the statement, and say it to her." You can hear a pin drop at that point. I encourage them to do it in spite of their anxiety. I promise that there is a point. "Mary, you are a fat disgusting blob." "Anne, your stomach is as large as your butt." Around the room we continue. The energy in the room is dense and dark. Then we process. What was that like? Why wasn't it funny saying it to someone else?

This is what you are doing to yourself multiple times a day. Your negative self-talk has the same dismal effect on your psyche. If you would not say something to your best friend, you should not be saying it to yourself. Indeed, most of us would not talk like this to a stranger or our worst enemy.

Maybe you do not realize the power of your negative thoughts. I encourage you to wake up and start replacing them with positive or at least more neutral talk. Depression and anxiety often accompany self-hate. These negative feelings can fuel yet more binge eating. Put simply, self-hate will sabotage your recovery.

This doesn't mean that we don't take responsibility for our screw ups. We shall fall and often. But it means we switch from an attitude of criticism to one of curiosity. Through gentle inquiry we can rewire our negative neural patterns. We can observe and learn from our mistakes, and finally we can get off this merry-go-round of disordered eating.

I hope you are beginning to understand how important it is to re-frame and change self-deprecating talk even if at first it feels like you are just changing words. Why? Because life can be painful enough. Because if you are like many with disordered eating, you feel things deeply. Because losing someone you love or getting a bad grade or losing a job challenges the best of us. Our negative self-talk adds insult to injury, making our already tenuous ability to cope with our emotions less and less likely.

The Three Voices of Compulsive Eating

Typically, there are three recognizable voices to compulsive eating. It is important to learn to recognize them all in order to strengthen one and weaken the other two.

1. **The "critic."** This is the main voice of the disorder. It may be similar to the voice of a person who criticized you in the past. Many of my clients call this part "ED" for eating disorder. Call this part whatever feels right, start recognizing it, and call it out. Apologize to yourself when you catch the critic being derogatory. Better yet, redo the statement in a kinder, gentler, or at least more neutral way.

"Fat talk" is connected to the critic as well. Fat talk is when we disparage ourselves or have a horrid day because we "feel fat" or bloated or our pants are tight. Just as we are learning that food is a symptom of a larger problem, we are also learning that fat talk or bad body thoughts are a symptom of something else. A mentally healthy individual has a wide range of emotions, but when we get caught in this cycle of self-criticism, eventually everything gets translated into the language of food, fat, and body image. So rather than feel sadness, we eat. Rather than realize what is really going on, we are just having a "fat" day.

2. **Hell with it.** For lack of a better term, I call the second voice, which is common in overeaters, the "Hell with it" voice. It is the part of you that despite the critic's admonishment, says that overeating this does

not matter. When you find yourself feeling compulsive, Hell with it says, "That's okay. Screw it. You need this NOW! You deserve it!" Of course, as soon as you eat or binge, the critic will be waiting. Hence, the vicious cycle.

Imagine being a parent and treating a child this way. The parent calls the child names, routinely underfeeds her and then encourages her to go ahead and eat whatever she wants. However, after she does, the parent calls her names again. How sad would that be? How would that child feel about themselves? Would such a child be confident? Of course not. And the effect is the same on you.

3. **The healthy voice**. This is the voice I call the self-mothering voice. It is our intuitive voice of wisdom. It is the most silent of the three voices when we are into our addictive eating patterns. Yet, it is the one we need the most. I have come to believe that recovery is, in part, a spiritual process. All addictions, including food, are destructive to both the body and the spirit. Since we often get caught up in the denial inherent to all addictions, this may come as a surprise. But the reality is that as we feed our addiction, we starve our spirit. Recovery will help us reconnect with our healthy voice. Through the use of SOFT AIM, we will learn a great deal about this voice and how to tap into it.

More on Diets

Part of the problem with diets is that they are born from our bad body image and our guilt and shame about food and weight. But, we will never shame ourselves into health and wellness. While committing to a diet may help us feel temporarily better, it is usually short lived. That renewed resolve and sense of control will crumble to shame and sadness with yet another failed promise to self. And where does that sense of shame lead us? More binging followed by yet another diet.

We also can acknowledge that we were never given the correct operating instructions. We live in a fat-phobic, thinness obsessed society. We may chase a weight that was only appropriate when we were in high school or be so restrictive we eventually start a pattern of binging. Women come in all shapes and sizes, yet we are told only one type of body is permissible. Jean Kilbourne in *Killing Us Softly: Advertisings Image of Women* says that only 5% of women naturally have the body type that the rest of us are expected to have.[6] The ideal is very tall and very lean, with long legs and large breasts. To make this even more daunting, you are either born with this body or not. And even the tall girls have problems. Most women who are naturally tall and long-legged have smaller breasts. It is the pear shaped girls who tend to have the larger breasts. So even when you see that model body, it has usually undergone surgical augmentation.

As you read earlier, diets have a high failure rate, yet they are given as the only tool for compulsive eating. If you are overweight, you may well have dieted your way to this weight. Diets not only can damage our metabolism, but they are also correlated with learning to binge and thus gaining more weight.

There are numerous benefits of recovery from disordered eating. If I did not believe this, I would not have written this book. Weight loss may be one of the side effects of your recovery. A diet, on the other hand makes us dependent on a scale, an external piece of metal that, in my experience, has too much power over most women. Diets give us weight loss tunnel vision. A diet makes weight loss or gain the SOLE focus. The reality is that weight is often a symptom of a bigger problem. Dieting and its singular goal of weight loss keep us from looking within. We stay focused on an external. Recovery is a focus on the internal.

Diets require that we put our life on hold until we arrive at the goal weight or can fit into the right pair of jeans. Few things that make me more regretful than the women, myself included, who have wasted years, indeed decades, putting their lives on hold. And guess what? Reaching goal weight is not the answer to everything wrong in our lives. Many can attest to having the same problems regardless of jean size.

If you picked up this book, you have probably figured out that your compulsive eating is about so much more than food, weight and body image. I wrote earlier about the fact that we cannot hate ourselves into recovery. Indeed, I say we must find our own healthy voice of compassion to recover. And remember, compulsive eating works in a sense. At that moment when we are drowning in emotion, it seems to ground us. Trouble is, it does nothing to problem solve or foster personal development. Binging just numbs us while our feelings are still stuffed down.

Honor what you have done to take care of yourself and honor the new path you are embarking on. I cannot guarantee that recovery will make you fit in your skinny jeans or hit your goal weight. I can, however, tell you that if you commit to this process, you will experience a sense of peace and well-being that yo-yo dieting and binging will not afford you.

Journal Assignment

1. It is time to practice paying attention to how compulsive eating operates in you. Notice factors such as how, why, when, and where you eat? How does your day go if your pants are tight? How does it go if they are loose? What is your inner dialogue?

2. Do you give yourself permission to make mistakes?

3. Do you believe you are worthy of recovery? Do you deserve to make peace with food and your body? Why or why not? If the answer is no, are you willing to explore this?

4. Notice how you are talking to yourself. Apologize when it is out of line. Put your self-talk in second person to assure you hear it clearly. Remember, if you would not say it to someone else, it is not okay to say it to yourself. Identify the voices of your disordered eating. Notice the critic. Identify your "Hell with it" voice. Most importantly FIND your healthy voice. Welcome it home.

CHAPTER 3

Letting Your Hunger Guide You

Eat when you are hungry. Sleep when you are tired.
                                                    -Old Zen Saying

Before we learn about SOFT AIM, our coping strategy for recovery, we have to get our eating under some semblance of structure. That is what this and the next chapter is about. I metaphorically call this stage the "bones" of recovery. These guidelines will help you build a foundation for recovery. I am asking you to hang in there because they may sound intimidating at first.

*** Important note: If you have been diagnosed with anorexia or have been very restrictive for some time, you may not feel physical hunger and you may feel full very quickly. These are some of the effects of starvation on the body. The hunger signal turns off and fullness happens too quickly. If this is the case, your binging (assuming you are binging) is likely a normal response to restriction. This chapter and the next (Enough Already) are not for you, not yet. Rather, you need a dietician versed in eating disorders to help you devise an appropriate meal plan. Your hunger will most likely return as you become healthier. Your satiety signal will likely normalize as well. Only at that point, is it appropriate to use hunger and satiety to guide you.

Recovery Guideline #1:

- *Eat when you are physically hungry.*

This sounds simple, but, lest we confuse simple with easy, allow me to explain. Simple and easy are two different matters when it comes to recovery. It is a simple concept that is hard to do.

Perhaps it doesn't sound simple to you but maybe it sounds crazy, simplistic, impossible or even revolutionary. I have had women express anger or fear when initially given this idea. Time and again I hear women say, "I just like food." Some will argue, "That's how I got into this mess." Others will complain, "But I'm always hungry." The fact of the matter is that overeating is NOT about liking food and physical hunger does not cause disordered eating. Actually, binging undermines the enjoyment and pleasure of food. It is in eating when we are hungry that we receive true pleasure in and gratitude for food. Maybe that first cookie or two in a binge is good, but not so much the rest of the batch. We seek the comfort of numbness when we binge, not the joy of good food.

Maybe you are afraid of your hunger. Maybe you think it has no end. Maybe you think you will devour the world with that hunger of yours. Maybe you think you don't deserve to eat. Maybe you don't trust your body. Maybe the countless diets and calorie counters and rules have left you suspicious of your hunger, the most obvious guideline for recovery.

I am not being naive. I am well aware that the reasons for disordered eating are much more involved and complex than just eating when you are hungry. But nonetheless, this is where you must start. You have to get back to the innate wisdom of your body. The body that will actually tell you when you are physically hungry. Since you have been taught to ignore your hungers for so long, you may find this idea frightening at first.

Believe it or not, physical hunger is something that you knew when you were a baby or small child. You also recognized when you

19

had eaten enough. You can learn this again. Hunger is a physiological mechanism. It is a birthright. For whatever multitude of reasons, you have lost biological hunger as the cue for when to eat. Eating when you are hungry is natural. Eating when you are NOT hungry is like scratching an itch that is not there. It is like peeing when you don't have to. It is like wanting to sleep when you are not tired. Your body will tell you when to eat just like it tells you when you need to use the restroom. You may be so out of touch with this cue, however, that relearning it will take some practice.

Learning to listen to your body's hunger signals will help you with other things as well. First, it is hard to focus on the emotional reasons for disordered eating until you end the maddening cycle of grazing or restricting all day and binging all night. Don't expect to be able to do this perfectly. No one does anything close to perfect with any of these principles.

Stepping out of the cycle of binging and restricting this little bit will give you the opportunity to identify some of the emotional reasons for your disordered eating. In addition, eating when you are hungry will be a reliable way to organize your eating. Eating out of physical hunger is the most clear cut way of telling you when you are not eating for the right reason. For every time you desire food when you are not physically hungry, there is something emotionally wrong. Ultimately, your job is to figure out what that is.

Remember we said earlier that food is not like an addiction to alcohol or drugs where complete abstinence is possible. Your hunger is actually the guidepost that will tell you when you need to eat. Your job, for now, is to ask yourself when you are reaching for food, if you are physically hungry. And regardless of the answer or the outcome, do not beat yourself up. Every time you are hard on yourself about this process, you extend the length of time recovery will take. Learning to eat in this natural way is also the beginning of good self-care.

One way to help you learn to properly gauge your physical hunger is a hunger measurement scale. The one below is similar to the one I used early in my own recovery. If you do an internet search, you can find many different versions of a measurement scale. Pick your favorite and use it until this concept becomes second nature and you can rate your hunger by the number without looking at this scale.

---

1 2 3 4 5 6 7 8 9 10

1-Starving, shaky, desperate, willing to eat almost anything. You will likely overeat from this place.
2-Very hungry, stomach growling, uncomfortable
3-Hungry, some physical sensation, stomach growling, feeling of emptiness, ready to eat.
4-Getting hungry. Almost there
5-Neither hungry nor satiated.
6-Satiated and satisfied. A physical signal of "enough" has sounded
7-Full. Slightly uncomfortable
8-More full. More uncomfortable
9-Really uncomfortable
10-Stuffed and very uncomfortable. This is how most of us feel after a binge.

I know...I know. You have a million reasons why this will not work. I don't have time to eat at work. I am not hungry until late, and it is bad to eat late. I am not hungry for breakfast. What if I am hungry and there is not any food? What if I am NOT hungry, but everyone is eating? What if there is something wonderful being served, but I am not hungry?

Let's start with the first one. Consider the following scenario: I don't have time to eat at work or school or whatever. One of the things we learn with intuitive eating is that sometimes we have to "manipulate" our hunger. Let's say you have scheduled dinner at a restaurant with family, but the reservation is not until 7 p.m. and you know you will be too hungry by then. On the scale, you predict you would likely be a #1 or #2. By the time the food arrives, definitely a

#1. Remember that being very hungry is a vulnerability. You will be more likely to overeat if you allow yourself to get this hungry. One of the things to do in this situation is to eat a snack when you recognize you are a #3 or #4 on the scale (hungry or almost hungry). Eat just enough to get yourself to a #5 on the scale, which is neither hungry nor satiated. In this way, you will likely be appropriately hungry by the time the food arrives.

Another challenge to eating when you are hungry is an overeater's fear that there will never be another chance to have a particular food. The offer of delectable food when you are not hungry is likely to produce a range of emotions. There is often a sense of loss, sadness, or even panic. You fear this may be the only opportunity to enjoy this food and you don't want to miss out. Truthfully, that is rarely the case. There will always be another opportunity for a cupcake or Italian food.. Truthfully, that is rarely the case. There will always be another opportunity for a cupcake or Italian food. Part of recovery, however, is expanding your self-care. You need to promise yourself that whatever you are NOT indulging in, you will eat when you *are* hungry. And you need to make good on your promises.

One of the things I really like about learning to identify and eat according to physical hunger is that sometimes you get to eat! This can be enjoyable for many reasons. Not only does food taste fantastic when you are hungry, but for many of us it is the first time in a long time that we do not feel guilty about the act of eating. Although food is required to live, many of us feel guilty every time we put food into our mouths.

Remember...even "normal" eaters overeat on occasion. The difference is they do not beat themselves up over it. They don't try to restrict to make up for it. They just wait until they are hungry to eat again.

Another scenario that can produce feelings of loss or panic is when you know you have had enough food, but you want to take more. For example, if there are three pieces of pizza left and you are satiated you know you should stop eating. The internal dialogue might run something like this: "But if I don't finish this off now, some-one else will. I may want it later, but it will be gone." This situation creates a sense of loss, of lack. The underlying fear is there is never enough. And that connects with the fear that "I" am not enough.

Why do you fear that there will not be enough for you? Why do you think you are not enough? The reasons are likely complex. I am reminded of one of my favorite sayings: "How you do anything is how you do everything." Compulsive overeaters tend to be more concerned about not having enough money or stuff. They tend to ac-cumulate more clutter, be it on their body or in their house.

Learning to eat when you are hungry will help you figure out the emotional underpinnings of your compulsive eating, and may even help you to become aware of what it is that you are truly hungry for. I am not talking about food. I am talking about a half-life, one that has been measured by calories, evolving into a full life. I am talking about exchanging that half-life for a life full of passion and goals and a full range of emotions.

How did we get so emotionally hungry? There are a myriad of reasons for emotional hunger; don't worry if you do not know what they are. Your hungers are likely very old and complex. Typically we hunger for things like connection, acceptance and creativity.

Recovery Guideline #2:

- *Drop the Diet Rules and Eat What You Want.*

At this point in recovery, it is essential that you drop the diet rules that have invaded your consciousness. This includes what you choose to eat. As long as you are hungry, anything goes. Now if you are dia-betic, have food allergies, Celiac disease, high cholesterol, or any other health issue, common sense must prevail. Harming yourself is never a good idea. But that said, if you have been a chronic dieter, you may crave things that are not considered "healthy." If you are taking the time to wait for physical hunger to eat, it is important you give yourself what you want. If you crave a hot creamy soup but tell yourself you have to eat a cold, crunchy salad, you will likely, after eating the salad, return to the kitchen for a night long grazing fiasco. Why? Because you were not emotionally satisfied. In the long run, the soup would have been a healthier choice because it did not lead to binging.

It may often be harder than soup vs. salad. I had a client eat a chocolate cake at least two meals a day for a week straight. She ate it when she was hungry, but after about a week, she lost all desire for it. Geneen Roth in her groundbreaking book, *Breaking Free from Compulsive Eating,* describes eating chocolate chip cookies whenever hunger called for several days.[1]

Why is it important that you drop the good food versus bad food belief? Because rebellion and self-sabotage are unfortunate obstacles on this path. If you are eating from hunger and eating what you want, there is less to rebel against. You have to take the thrill out of forbidden foods. If you are like most compulsive overeaters, you have likely been on so many diets that just the slightest suspicion of more deprivation will elicit a rebellious full out binge. Eventually, when the little kid in you realizes you are all done with deprivation, your feelings of rebellion will lessen. You may actually start to crave healthier foods or more balanced meals. I have seen many women who embraced this concept eventually find ways to change their eating to more healthy choices without the binging and self-sabotage. But in the meantime, if you are hungry and eating what you want, you are likely eating less food, even if what you eat is a decadent dessert.

Other diet rules to let go:

- Don't eat after 7 p.m.
- Eat according to blood type
- Eat only certain combinations of food
- Don't eat carbohydrates
- Don't eat white sugar or flour
- Only eat "healthy" food

Not only do you need to eat when you are hungry, you need to be mindful that you are doing so. For years I would match eating lunch with *The Young and The Restless*. And because the program lasted an hour, my lunch took an hour. That is a lot of eating. Part of the reason I kept eating was I was oblivious to the first bites. I was distracted.

If you wait until you are hungry to eat and plan on stopping when you are satiated, you need to minimize distractions so you can be mindful and enjoy eating. Food tastes better when you are hungry. Indeed, it actually tastes like something. You can better enjoy the aroma and textures of food when you are hungry. You can and should eat with gusto and pleasure.

This is as good a time as any to offer a few other suggestions that will help you own and honor your physical hunger. First, eat in full view of others. No, I don't expect those of you who live alone to eat only at restaurants. I am talking about the other stunts you likely pull to hide your eating. These include things like eating in the car, waiting until your loved ones leave the house to binge, throwing away the wrappers (aka evidence). I think I have used or heard a client admit every trick imaginable. No more hiding. If you are hungry, you deserve to be fed. You, like any other adult human, have the right to choose what you are going to feed yourself. I know that this may cause issues with well-meaning family members. You may need to have an honest talk with any loved one that is apt to comment on your eating or food choices.

Back to eating without distraction. That means not only no television but no eating while driving a car. There may be a time when you can be more lenient on this but it will help immensely if you, when you are finally hungry, stay as mindful of what you are doing as possible. It comes down to this. Imagine you are following through with this plan. You are not eating until you are appropriately hungry. The moment is here. You are a #3 on the hunger scale. The pizza has arrived. If you are not mindful, if you are watching your favorite show, you will miss the joy of eating. You will not taste the food. It will be over in a flash. You will not recognize when you have had enough.

Another thing that sabotages success is having emotionally intense or tension filled eating experiences. Digestion slows when you are upset, making it more difficult to know how much food is enough. The addiction recovery movement uses an acronym titled, "HALT." It stands for hungry, angry, lonely, and tired; it reminds individuals that these four issues are triggers for relapse. When they show up, it is time to "halt" and pay attention. For compulsive eaters, getting too hungry is a trigger for overeating. In terms of the hunger scale, you want to avoid getting to a #1 or a #2. It will be very difficult not to overeat if you do.

The length of time that this aspect of recovery will take varies by individual. It will be difficult for some to find their physical hunger but with practice it will come. Your hunger will guide you back home to yourself every time. It is up to you to let it.

Practice

When you are hungry, ask yourself what you want. Trust the wisdom of your body. Your hunger is your compass. Don't worry about what you choose. You have to start where you are. Remember, you need to convince your beaten down self that you are done with self-loathing and restriction. Give yourself what you want. Eliminate distractions. Taste the food, chew it, enjoy it and finally, write about it.

Journal Assignment

1. What are some of the issues/obstacles that interfere with your ability to eat when you are hungry?
2. How do you know when you are hungry?
3. Are you aware of what is enough?
4. Do you let yourself eat when you are hungry?
5. How do you decide when it is time to eat?
6. What are your diet rules? How hard will it be to unlearn them?
7. What reaction are you having to the recovery guideline of eating when you are hungry and eating what you want?
8. What in your life are you really hungry for? What do you need? What do you yearn for? Do not edit yourself. Just write.

CHAPTER 4

Enough Already

Come back to yourself. Return to the voice of the body. Trust yourself.

-Geneen Roth

Recovery Guideline #3:

- *Stop eating when you are satisfied.*

This chapter will be about combining eating when you are hungry with stopping when you are satisfied. I won't lie. Figuring out when you are physically hungry is usually easier than stopping when you are satisfied. We may also fear that we will never stop eating which makes it even harder to know what is enough. We may have become so used to the pain of overeating that we are frightened if we do not feel at least a slight discomfort when we leave the plate. We have been taken so far from the innate wisdom of our body that this notion of "enough" is suspect. We have waged battle on our natural hunger and appetites and satiety for a multitude of reasons and rules. This suggestion to stop eating when your body tells you to, may seem impossible.

But believe it or not, there was a time when you knew how to do this. Eating when hungry and stopping when satisfied is something that nearly all mammals are programmed to do from birth. Yet many of us have lost this ability. The "norm" is to eat until we are at least slightly uncomfortably full. Many cultures actually discourage this, suggesting one push away from food while there is still room.

Allowing our body to tell us when it has had enough means we leave the eating experience with mental acuity. No more feeling foggy and uncomfortable and needing a nap. We will likely have more energy to do something. Stopping at satiety also means we actually feel better at the end of a meal. Imagine that. Not numb and physically uncomfortable, but better.

Even if being overly full has been your normal, it wasn't always that way. Up until about age five, you likely had an innate awareness of your hunger, crying for food when you were hungry and ignoring it when you were full. You were guided by your hormones, namely ghrelin and leptin. Levels of ghrelin, a hormone that regulates hunger, rise when your body needs food; leptin, often called the satiety hormone, is triggered when you're satiated. We have to reconnect with the internal signal provided by leptin to tell us when to stop eating. This is another one of the reasons we need to eat without distraction. It is already hard enough to hear the signal. The distractions we talked about in the last chapter (television blaring, driving, difficult conversations, etc.) only make it that much harder. We have to slow down in order to figure out this part. And it may take a while.

Just to make this concept trickier, the signal that tells us we have had enough only "pings" once. The one diet rule I have come to accept as fact is that it takes about 20 minutes for the signal to reach the brain. And thus, you need to eat mindfully and slowly and without distraction to hear this voice. It is not realistic to assume you will always be able to eat without distraction. Life is more complicated than that. But the more you practice now, the sooner you will learn to hear the ping that signals enough.

One reason hearing your satiety cue and stopping can be hard is that you may have an "all or none" relationship with food. This may make last week's assignment of eating when you are hungry difficult as well. You have been deprived for so long that once you start eating, you can barely stop. This is where diets and restriction have caused more problems. Your body reads hunger as famine and you feel compelled to gorge yourself as a survival instinct. So, when alas, you finally eat, it is not only your emotions but your physiology that takes over. Your body innately is driven to over fill before yet another food draught ensues.

The Key's Semi-starvation Study illustrates how the body reacts to starvation.[1] The study was not conducted as part of eating disorder research but was conducted after World War II to study how to refeed starving war victims. In this study, Keys and his colleagues recruited young men who had no eating disorder or body image issues. These were just average guys who were considered both physically and psychologically healthy. What was astounding was that after these men were put on a low calorie diet similar to the ones that many women routinely live on, they started experiencing alarming symptoms. All of the subjects became obsessed with food. Their metabolism plummeted. They were irritable, tired, and depressed. When given the chance, they binged. When the refeeding time of the experiment began, they had a great deal of trouble recognizing satiety. They continually over-ate. It took them months to learn normal hunger signals again. And remember, these were men who had no body image issues. They had no cultural ideal that they were aspiring to. These were regular guys.

If you've been ignoring your hunger and fullness signals for a long time, you too may have temporarily lost your physical sensitivity to hunger and/or fullness. This is often the outcome of years of dieting and restricting food. You may also have been raised as part of the "clean your plate" club, having parents that encouraged you to finish all your food whether you were still hungry or not. If this is the case for you, it will take some time to rediscover hunger and fullness cues. And remember, if you have trouble with this, be kind and be patient with yourself. It will take a while.

Sometimes, eating according to hunger and satiety is frightening because it involves being connected to your body. If you have been abused or in any way fear experiencing your emotions, you may have blocked out many of your physiological sensations. The rest of this book and understanding SOFT AIM will help you to reconnect. Getting a therapist of your own would be beneficial as well.

Interestingly, lack of sufficient sleep makes it difficult to hear both hunger and satiety signals. Many of us run on empty and are consistently sleep deprived. We now understand that too little sleep causes an increase of ghrelin which in turn increases hunger. In addition, too little sleep lowers the production of leptin which tells us when we have eaten enough.[2]

To make matters worse, some overeaters may be leptin-resistant. This seems to be more likely in obese individuals who have chronically dieted. But don't despair. Even if you are truly leptin-resistant, it does not have to be permanent. The last thing you want to do is restrict more by going on another low calorie diet. This will lower your ability to hear fullness signals further and slow your metabolism to a stop. Eating regular meals and eating according to cues of physical hunger are good places to start healing any hormone imbalances.

If you have trained your body to ignore hunger signals, you have likely trained it to ignore fullness signals as well.

Practical Tips to know if you are Satiated

- Go back and look at the hunger scale from the last chapter.
- Make sure you are appropriately hungry when you start eating. Remember, this is about a 3 on the hunger scale. Be sure you are eating something you desire. If you aren't, it will be even more difficult for you to feel satisfied.
- Eat slowly. Your meal should take at least 20 minutes. Again, that is how long it takes to know if you are satiated. If you are racing along, you will miss the cue.

- Put down your fork between bites. Breathe.
- Eat without distraction and avoid difficult conversations. There will be a time when it is okay to watch television or read while eating, but not until this is second nature.
- Savor and taste each bite. Give thanks for how the food came to your table. Notice the colors and textures. Think of the nutrients. Make eating a sacred experience.
- When you think that maybe you have eaten the right amount of food to satisfy you without the pain of over fullness, ask yourself if you can stop eating.

Some people feel a sense of sadness and loss when their meal is over. If stopping is something you can do, put down the fork. Set a timer for 10-15 minutes. Remember, this is not your last meal. You can eat whenever you are hungry. If you are still hungry when the timer goes off, you can go back for more. This is very important. You are working to regain your self-trust. You have to feed yourself. You deserve to feed your physical hunger.

If you find yourself unable to stop and do indeed overeat to the point of discomfort, you need to forgive yourself. All is not lost. Just wait until you are physically hungry again to eat. Maybe you will not be hungry for the snack you planned on eating or the next meal will need to be later than you planned. That Is okay. It is very important that you simply learn to listen to the cues of your body to eat.

A good goal is to remain around that 3-6 range on the hunger and satiety scale. Much less than 3 and you will be too hungry. As you go up the scale toward 10, you will be increasingly uncomfortable. Know too that your stomach is like an expandable bag. As you eat smaller meals and snacks, your stomach will adjust to the smaller portions, and you will feel satisfied more quickly. If you start eating when you are not hungry, you will never know what is enough. Remember, emotional hunger is never satisfied.

Finally, trust that your body is innately capable...listen. This is about taking your power back. Perhaps for the first time in a long time, you are letting your body guide you.

- You decide what to eat.
- You decide how much.
- You decide if you like it.
- You decide when you've had enough.

You just need to slow down and stop overriding the signals. It is time to listen.

Personally, one of the main gifts of the first three guidelines--eating from hunger, eating what you want and stopping when you have had enough--is that once you start trusting your body, the benefits multiply. We recognize thirst as a reason to get a drink of water. Your body wants to rest, you rest. It wants to move, you move. You are tired, you sleep. When sad, you cry. When you decide someone seems ill suited for you or a situation no longer fits, you don't plod desperately along afraid to say no. Once you start listening to the wisdom of your body, the whispers get more audible. You need only to listen.

The Eventual Ideal

Ideally, (and please note the word "ideally") when you start eating and stop eating based on internal signals, you will begin to average three to six eating experiences a day. Specifically, that translates to the following:

> Breakfast
> Post-breakfast snack
> Lunch
> Afternoon snack
> Dinner
> Post-dinner snack

I can hear you now. "Six times a day? I will definitely gain weight!" Let me explain. The typical overeater is a restrictor by day and a binger by night. I know the drill. I did it for years. I started out renewed each day. Renewed often meant skipping breakfast, having a wrap or low calorie frozen dinner and diet coke for lunch. When I arrived home I was both physically starved, and emotionally depleted, I would eat my way through the evening. I did this only to wake up the next morning guilty and ashamed; then I'd repeat the cycle. Get the picture? Many of you, I know, are living this script. It gets old. It gets exhausting. It is spiritually and emotionally deadening. It is hard to feel good about yourself when you break a promise to yourself on a daily basis. But you are set up to fail by this cycle. Despite all of your best efforts, your body is driven to make up for the daily deficit. This drive, exacerbated by a hard day and the demands of the evening, is too much to overcome. You need to balance out your day. Your recovery will depend on it.

The Breakfast Contradiction

You must eat breakfast. Just when you thought you were figuring things out, I throw this in. And it contradicts the entire, "Eat when you are hungry" rule. Remember, I told you this was an imperfect path. Anyway, you need to eat breakfast every morning hungry or not. This is the only meal to which this contradiction applies. If you miss breakfast, the cycle is more likely to continue. Once you binge at night, you are even less likely to want breakfast because you are still full from the night before. You must eat breakfast to start a new recovery day. You must eat breakfast to avoid that heavy calorie load that has likely become the end of the day norm.

And remember, eating six times is the "ideal" scenario. The fact is, you will likely get hungry every few hours if you are eating when you are hungry and stopping when satiated. This averages out to six eating experiences a day. That said, you do not need to march lock-step to this part of recovery. If you eat too much at a meal, (which is likely at the beginning of recovery) you may not be hungry for a snack. Just be certain to do the breakfast part. Your goal is to stop eating in time to be hungry again for a snack or a meal in a few hours. And believe it or not, I am not going to suggest that you start "food-logging" all of this. It will be more helpful, if you are willing, to create a chart and simply check if you ate breakfast, lunch, dinner or any of the three snacks. Just a check and a hunger and satiety number. For example, breakfast may look like this:

B (for Breakfast)	Hunger/Satiety level
X	4/7

In the above example, the "x" indicates that breakfast was eaten and your hunger level started at 4 and you were at a 7 when you finished. Remember, you are not concerned with what you ate or how big the portion was. Even though you have finished Chapter One, about becoming conscious of your disordered eating and changing your negative self-talk, you are still working on that concept every day. By waiting until you are hungry and stopping when you are not, you are learning more about how compulsive eating behavior works in you.

It is important that you not beat yourself up for your struggles with these aspects of recovery. Remember, this is about much more than food. You have been trying the best you could to take care of yourself through overeating. You have to practice compassion or you will be stuck in self-loathing forever. Don't look now, but you are also making peace with your body and your hunger. Instead of hating and trying to control your hunger and your body, you are lovingly taking care of yourself. You are learning to listen to your innate wisdom. It was always there. You just stopped listening.

Do not for a minute underestimate how radical your recovery is. Our culture is obsessed with thinness. It tells us in a million ways that our bodies and most definitely our hungers cannot and should not be trusted. Rather, they should be starved, toned, controlled, stuffed into clothes that don't fit, and surgically altered if necessary. We are told that we must attain thinness no matter the cost. And here you are, reading a book and embarking on a path that simply tells you to eat what you want when you are hungry. It is nothing less than revolutionary.

Journal Assignment

1. Are you practicing eating when you are hungry and stopping when you are satisfied? What is that like for you?
2. What is it like to eat what you want? What feelings does that bring up in you?
3. What do you think of the idea of eating three meals and three snacks and matching those to hunger and satiety?
4. How do you normally decide to stop eating?
5. **Practice:** Try matching your hunger and satiety to three meals and three snacks. Write about your successes and struggles.

CHAPTER 5

SOFT AIM

Knowing yourself is the beginning of all wisdom.

-Aristotle

Let's review what we have learned so far:

- Become aware of and challenge any negative self-talk.
- Recognize the three voices of disordered eating: The critic, Hell with it, and the healthy self-mothering voice.
- Recognize physical hunger as the cue for eating.
- Eat what you want when you are hungry.
- Learn what amount of food your body needs to become satiated but not overly full.

Now it is time to talk about SOFT AIM, an important tool that will offer you support in the moments of craving and times of distressing emotions. SOFT AIM is an acronym for the seven steps in this strategy. It directs your attention during what, for overeaters, is often a difficult time. The process can be practiced in writing, although once you have practiced SOFT AIM, you can perform the process automatically without the need to write anything down. I have used SOFT AIM with clients, and I make it a regular practice of my own. The seven steps of the strategy of SOFT AIM are as follows:

SOFT AIM:
S-STOP
O-Observe
F-Feelings
T-Thoughts
A-Allow
I-investigate
M-Mother

If this does not seem clear, do not be concerned. The following chapters will explain each letter of the acronym and how each letter corresponds to a step in your recovery process. SOFT AIM is a tool that will help you to slowly unravel the emotional drivers that lead to overeating. More importantly, it will help you develop the third voice in the trio you learned from Chapter 2: the healthy voice. Practiced regularly, SOFT AIM will help you to know yourself better. As Aristotle said in the above quote, *"Knowing yourself is the beginning of all wisdom."* Before I go into the strategy of SOFT AIM, let's talk a little about stress and our brain.

Our Nervous System

The "starve and binge" pattern that many women engage in has an effect on the body. Time and again, I hear women express fear about how unhealthy they are at their current weight. But rarely do they consider that constant worry and distress about weight can, in itself, have a profound negative effect on both their psychological and physical well-being.

Our nervous system is comprised of the parasympathetic and sympathetic nervous system. The parasympathetic nervous system is commonly called the relaxation response. It quiets the mind and relaxes the body. The sympathetic nervous system is our fight/flight/freeze response. It is a primal response that has ensured our survival from predators and life threatening danger. Unfortunately, the body cannot distinguish between a saber tooth tiger and someone taking your parking space. And when the body is in the fight/flight/flee mode, it does not have time to handle any little cancer cells or cold germs that come up. Our immune system becomes suppressed. No repairing or healing can happen. It does not matter if you drink green juice or go to the gym. In addition, there is a host of other maladies associated with the stress response: headaches, gastrointestinal issues and asthma. As you can see, we are not doing ourselves any favors by engaging in the constant, "Oh my GOD. I have to lose weight NOW!" war.

Think of the sympathetic nervous system as a team of paramedics. If they are coming to rescue you from a serious accident, they are not worried about treating a cold germ or a hang nail. Everything else has to take the back seat for your survival. Overuse of the stress response keeps you in an unhealthy survival mode. Scientists have learned that hormonally you are less likely to lose weight when you are stressed because cortisol is flooding our bodies, and undermining our efforts.[1] SOFT AIM teaches us to relax and stay in the present moment. Aiming, but softly. No force or stress. That is where true recovery happens.

By using the skills of SOFT AIM for recovery, you are strengthening your prefrontal cortex.[2] You do this by coming back to the present moment, by demonstrating self-compassion, and by questioning unhealthy thoughts. In this way the prefrontal cortex can better regulate your overactive amygdala and the revving up or shutting down response of the nervous system. Due to early trauma, many of us developed an overactive amygdala, and unfortunately did not develop the resiliency we need to properly manage stress. The prefrontal cortex is a handy part of our brain, capable of empathy, self-awareness, wise discernment and conscious reflection. It integrates two parts of the brain: the focusing network which concentrates on facts and the defocusing network which can link old ideas together in new ways. The prefrontal cortex weighs input from the logical left hemisphere with input from the intuitive right hemisphere. In short, this part of our brain needs to be strong and resilient.

Beyond the acronym, SOFT AIM describes the mindset you need to use as you approach recovery. You are aiming, but softly and gently. This means without judgment or force. This means putting aside the goal of losing weight. Letting weight loss be the side effect of recovery, not the goal.

Our culture, like most western societies, values and emphasizes striving and producing. Actually, we are pretty much obsessed with it. But some things can be better achieved with a softer focus. Why? Because the energy and anxiety of struggle get in the way of achievement. How do you "lean" into recovery? You need to accept where you are right now. You must focus on your behavior *now*.

This is a tricky concept to understand, so hang in there. SOFT AIM is similar to the Buddhist philosophy of non-striving. According to this philosophy, only when we stop fighting to reach our goal, can we start to see the "forest for the trees" or the "bigger picture." We cannot force recovery. The way we approach recovery through the SOFT AIM process is to drop judgment and our attachment to outcome.

How many times have you put conditions around recovery? You may think, "Well, I will try eating when I am hungry as long as I don't gain weight." Or "I will try this recovery thing after I lose weight." This creates anxiety that diminishes your progress. When it comes to recovery you need to be passionate AND mindful AND compassionate. You need to remember you are more than your body and your disordered relationship with food. You need to remember you are already good enough as you are. When you try to simply discipline ourselves into recovery, you cannot help but become harsh and perfectionistic. You give up. You wear down. This is another reason, diets, which rely on self-discipline alone, do not work.

Let's explore the subject of perfectionism. I would be astonished if your recovery resembled anything close to perfect. It is complex. You are complex. This is not a black and white issue. It, like most everything in this big complicated world, is gray. Food matters are especially gray. Food cannot be avoided. Recovery means that every few hours you face the object of your addiction. And most importantly, perfectionism does not work. It leads to more compulsive behavior, not less. How many times have you "broken" your diet and ridden right off the rails for the rest of the day, week, month or year? Perfectionism strikes again.

If you are like most compulsive eaters, you are not often mindful or in the moment. Think of binges. They are mindless. Binges are trance-like. You are not really tasting, you are lost. Dieting too, is not in the present. You are clawing your way toward the future when you will reach the "holy grail" also known as "goal weight." If you are aiming softly, you can be mindful and present in the here and now. Mindfulness is a fundamental principle of recovery.

Aiming softly can be understood in the light of parenting. We can set a goal, such as having a child that does not lie, cheat or steal. But no matter what we do, we cannot guarantee the outcome of that desire. We can, on the other hand, focus on teaching and modeling that behavior to our child in the present moment. It is the same with recovery. To reach our goal, we need to understand that we have limited control over the final outcome, but we do have complete control over our behavior right now.

How often have you gone on a diet and done really well, eating less, drinking water and exercising only to get on the scale to find out you have not lost a pound? For many of you, when that great oracle, commonly known as a scale, says that you have not lost weight, the diet is over. You TRIED, but when the scale is the grader, you will ultimately fail. If you want to succeed you need to drop your weight loss as a primary focus.

Psychologist Daniel Wegner explored what he called the "ironic effects" of effort.[3] For example, if I tell you not to think about a pink elephant, you probably will. If you try too hard to get back to sleep when you have insomnia, you will probably stay awake. Sometimes force has the opposite effect. This applies to recovery too. When we stop the war, we can recover.

Austrian psychologist Victor Frankl pioneered the comparable concept "paradoxical intention".[4] Used often in psychotherapy, paradoxical intention is similar to reverse psychology. It is the deliberate practice of a neurotic habit or thought, in order to reverse it. If someone has insomnia, they will be encouraged to stay awake. When instructed to stay awake, they will fall asleep faster.

When working with compulsive eaters, I often find myself telling my clients to eat more frequently and regularly. After a lifetime of being told to restrict, being told to eat can actually decrease the desire to binge. Compulsive eaters tend to eat too little during the day and save all their calories for evening which, as we have learned, is not a good idea. They must shift their focus from eating less (the typical diet approach) to eating enough and eating throughout the day. Back to those six eating experiences discussed in an earlier chapter. This is also a bit of paradoxical intention. Become more concerned that you eat enough rather than too much. By unwinding all of the ingrained diet rules, you will be able to work toward your goal more gently.

All that said, there will be times you need good old fashioned willpower. It is just that willpower alone will not sustain you through something this complex. You may need it at times to break your old habits, but it only lasts so long. Do you need evidence of this? Look at your long list of diets and diet failures. You can't live like that forever.

We, like all other living things, are organisms. And one thing that scientists know about organisms is that they are motivated by intention. Force however, creates fear and anxiety. We also know that fear contracts intention. So again, without embracing and relaxing into recovery through SOFT AIM, you keep spinning your wheels and end up back at the beginning. And why do you want to quiet your fear? Partly because it will be impossible to hear the healthy voice if you are rigidly chasing a number on a scale.

When, you may wonder, is willpower helpful? Allow me to provide an example from my own life. In the early days of my recovery, one of my bad habits was that when I walked in the door from work, I walked directly to the kitchen. I would find something, anything, to munch on. This behavior had nothing to do with hunger. It was my way of disconnecting from work and calming myself down. It was also the beginning of the night long binge that I was prepping for.

Willpower was what it took to walk past the kitchen and straight into the bedroom. I would get directly into the shower and wash off the day's stress. I would change into comfortable clothes. I would not enter the kitchen until I had a plan. This, however was not always the case. Sometimes I would walk in the kitchen, open the fridge and slam it, open the cupboard and slam it, walk out of kitchen, walk back into the kitchen, repeat. Sometimes I had to lock myself up in the bedroom, leave the house, and do whatever it took. And more times than I can count, I failed and binged anyway. When that happened, I was compassionate with myself. And I tried again and again. Dr. Kristen Neff, a prominent proponent of self-compassion says that while we think we need to beat ourselves up to stay on track and do better, the opposite is true. Self-compassion actually enhances our motivation and productivity.[5]

SOFT AIM means we accept we are in this for the long haul, for however long recovery may take. SOFT AIM means we are still here today regardless of our imperfection. SOFT AIM means we are living in the present moment. It means we are working on recovery by focusing on our behavior now. It is not giving up; it is giving up the force and the struggle. Ironically, the energy of peace draws us closer to what we want. The writer and teacher, Tosha Silver says, "The very act of grasping for the feather creates the wind current that pushes it away."[6] Not forcing your recovery, therefore, can help you to be more positive about it. Why? Because you are forgiving and compassionate with yourself. You are working on your recovery without focusing only on the finish line.

Speaking of finishing lines, you might be wondering what if your recovery has an end point. While I have seen people fully recover from disordered eating, it is possible that recovery will be a permanent part of your life. If so, is that okay? Can you relinquish attachment to an outcome? To weight goals, to jean size?

I understand that you probably want a perfect and complete recovery, but remember we live in a society of crazy people who are addicted to size. Even women without disordered eating, have body image issues. It is sometimes hard to know if we are finished or cured. Again, it is food. And maybe for you, how you handle food will always be a doorway to understanding what is going on in your life. It is just that when recovery is your goal, you will be aware when emotional triggers are driving your food intake.

When you embrace SOFT AIM, you are like an athlete who is in "the zone." Many articles have been written on this concept, and they all say basically the same thing: The zone is a mental state of total focus on the present moment. There is no worry about outcome, but there is a degree of self-trust. There is no "paralysis by analysis," and most important, there is no self-judgment.

Ways to Aim Softly

- Let go. Let God. Take a leap of faith. Trust the journey. Realize that recovery from disordered eating is bigger than you are. Give yourself up. If God does not feel like the right term to you, give yourself up to the universe, to life, to the present reality, or whatever works for you.
- Aim for the right thing. If you treat recovery like the "eat when you're hungry, stop when you're not diet," you will not achieve recovery. If you hate yourself, you will not achieve true recovery either. It will be counterfeit. It will not last. It will be just one more thing you tried and failed at. Simply do the next right thing.
- Let go of multi-tasking. Doing more than one thing at a time will scatter and drain your energy. It will also make it more difficult to remember to STOP (the first part of SOFT AIM) and to listen to the self-mothering voice (the last part).
- Practice mindfulness. You will learn more about this in subsequent chapters.
- If you want recovery, focus on your choices today, not long term outcomes.

- Stop *trying* to lose weight. It is like *"trying* to get it together, *trying* to clean the house or *trying* to wash the car." More often than not it does not happen. It separates you from taking responsibility for your food intake and recovery.

So, what exactly does SOFT AIM look like? Keep reading. The strategy is described through every letter in the acronym.

Journal Assignment

1. Which of the following might be barriers to embracing the SOFT AIM approach to recovery?
   - Other people's judgment
   - Fear of failure
   - Perfectionism
   - Fear of losing control
   - Low self-esteem and self-loathing
   - Impatience
   - Desire for a quick fix
   - Trying too hard
   - Wrong focus
   - Fear you will not be able to handle emotions without food.
   - Fear of weight gain

CHAPTER 6

Steady Now and Stop

> Learn to pause or nothing worthwhile will catch up to you.
>
> *-Doug King*

Stopping means that when we are in the moment of a craving or we are experiencing an uncomfortable emotion, we are able to pause and identify what is happening within us. It may sound easy or overly simplistic. Actually, I believe stopping may be the hardest part of SOFT AIM. Stopping may be the part of the process we forget 1000 times.

Stopping requires coming into the "now" of the moment. Not yesterday, not the future, but the "What the hell is going on right now?" moment. I could have called it "pausing" as well. We have all used the pause button on a remote control. Imagine yourself pressing pause when you feel the urge to compulsively eat. Giving yourself delay time is often a huge help. Most overeaters go straight from the urge to the behavior. Delaying buys us some well needed time. The truth is that cravings and compulsions do not last forever. They will pass if you can stop and turn off the auto-pilot that usually drives your disordered eating.

Why is this step so much harder than it sounds? Because again, our unhealthy thoughts are often automatic and run at a subconscious level. They are firmly entrenched in our psyche and usually learned by age six. They are not accustomed to being questioned. Stopping is very threatening and, therefore very hard to do. Scientist Bruce Lipton estimates 95% of our thoughts run at an unconscious level.[1] We are more or less running on auto-pilot. When we have a craving or feel an unsettling emotion, if food has been the drug we use to handle such challenges, our decision is made even before we get up and head to the kitchen. Lipton suggests that the 95% unconscious and 5% conscious awareness is too generous; only those who really work at conscious awareness have that 5%. For the others, it is more like 99% unconscious and 1% conscious.

Simply put, the unconscious mind is nothing more than the neural pathways of everything we have learned over the years. For most of us, that is a great deal of limiting beliefs, fears, and misguided perceptions. Just because you consciously recognize and want to change old patterns, does not in itself, change anything. You may know something consciously, but the subconscious brain will seek out experiences to prove that the old way is better. For example, if you believe that you cannot cope with negative emotions unless you calm yourself with food, your brain will seek to prove that.

Think of your unhealthy neural pathways as being like an old groove that a wheelbarrow has gone down countless times. You try to send the wheelbarrow down a new path, but it is much easier to fall into that well-worn groove. And just because you manage once or twice to send it down the new path, it doesn't mean that the trench has disappeared. It is still there and much stronger than the new path. It will take a great deal of practice and mindfulness to get the new neural pathway as strong as the old one. And still more practice to get it stronger than the old pathway.

You have to consciously choose to stop if you are going to cease using food for comfort and break the automatic behavior. If you do not, you will not be able to use the rest of SOFT AIM. You will not be able to think through or even recognize and understand your issues and problems. You will not have the time to honestly look at what the consequences of that next binge will be. You will not be able to make a mindful choice about your behaviors.

Stopping is the antithesis of compulsion. The last thing your craving wants you to do is stop. So again, that is why this is easier said than done and why it will take practice. You are acting contrary to your inner workings and wiring. Your consciousness is getting in the way of the desired outcome.

By stopping when you recognize a craving or uncomfortable feeling, you are taking the time to say you are important enough to do this work. You are breaking a well ingrained pattern and making an important paradigm shift.

Once again, while recovery may seem simple, it is not easy. It is a process as opposed to an event. Being compassionate with yourself is a must. Although you may fall many times, you need to get back up and practice again and again.

Daily Check-ins

Sometimes, when you're in the midst of a craving, you may feel that stopping is next to impossible. Another way to trick your brain into stopping is simply to slow everything down for the moment. Just imagine everything moving in slow motion. If you are typing, slow it down. Walking, slow it down. Talking, slow it down. You may be able to stop from that slowed down place more easily. Others find it helpful to imagine seeing a giant red STOP sign and hear themselves yell, "STOP!"

Regardless of how you go about it, the S in SOFT aim is something you want to practice doing when things are not so detrimental. While much of SOFT AIM is for dealing with and circumventing emotional eating, the moment of craving will of course be the hardest time to stop. Stop and check in with yourself throughout the day in order to build mindfulness. By practicing stopping, you are practicing awareness. This means you are starting to live more consciously and this will enable you to better regulate your thoughts and emotions. Meditating for 15-30 minutes a day will accelerate your healthy brain change. A practice of yoga may do the same. But do not despair. Most of us are not as great at meditation as we would like. Most of us have trouble finding the time. Most of us have minds like a circus show. It is okay to practice in small increments. This can be as simple as setting a timer for once an hour or once a day to simply pause and take a breath or two. Another helpful idea is to check in with yourself every morning, literally stop and check in.

Mindfulness Practices

One way to increase awareness is to find a mindfulness practice that is helpful to you. These are some of my favorites. Try them out. Write the one or ones you like best in your journal. Practice!

- Peace/Calm: On an inhale, mentally, say the word, "Peace." On the exhale, say the word "Calm". If your mind wanders, go back to the word "peace" or "calm." Try saying the word and breathing as slowly as possible. Do this three to five times. Voila! You stopped.
- Movement Meditation: Put your hands in prayer position at your chest. As you inhale slowly raise your hands (still in prayer position) up over your head. As you exhale, slowly bring them back to your chest. Repeat three to five times. End with palms open over heart, sending a message to yourself of self-love and peace.
- Body Awareness Meditation: Scan your body. Find a part that is not feeling tense. Focus all of your attention on that part of your body. For example, perhaps you pick your left elbow. For the purposes of this exercise, you would put all of your attention on feeling the life in your left elbow; feeling how your left elbow is attached to your body. This feeling may be a sensation of nerves or blood or bone.
- Another form of body awareness is to, "feel the life in your arms and legs." Years ago I went to a week-long retreat of Geneen Roth. Geneen has written several useful books on recovery. At the retreat, the facilitators repeatedly told us to stop and "Feel the life in your arms and legs."

- Notice where your hands touch this book or device. Notice where your feet make contact with the floor; notice their heaviness.
- Stop and notice your breath. Are you breathing in? Okay. Slowly breathe out. Are you breathing in? Okay. Slowly breathe out. Repeat for at least three to five breaths.
- Use any of your senses to ground and center. Close your eyes and try to identify three different sounds. Give yourself a hand massage with scented lotion which evokes the senses of both touch and smell.
- Journal. When you write, you are stopping and working to recognize your emotional state.

What is the point of the above exercises and why do they help us with the "Stop" of SOFT AIM? Both cravings and uncomfortable emotions activate the "fight or flight" response. Being mindful triggers the parasympathetic nervous system and helps counteract the sympathetic nervous system's "fight or flight" response. Over time, repeated practice of "stopping" and being mindful will strengthen the prefrontal cortex and weaken the connection to our overactive amygdala which warns us of danger. For many overeaters the amygdala acts like the character "Chicken Little" who is always proclaiming the sky is falling.

Stopping will be just that. You step out of the loop long enough to realize you are headed for the kitchen or another fast food drive through. You stop and ask, "What am I doing? What number am I on the hunger scale? Am I physically hungry?" If the answer to this last question is "Yes," carry on and feed yourself for goodness sake. If the answer is no, stop and breathe. Pick one of the above practices. At the very least take three slow breaths in and out. You have stopped. You have stepped out of your firmly entrenched, fear-based behavior pattern. You are in the present moment. You may wonder what you are to do after you stop. Read on; because this is where the rest of SOFT AIM comes in.

Journal Assignment

1. How will you implement daily check-ins into your recovery? Remember the S of SOFT AIM (STOPPING) will be easier to do if you have practiced pausing regularly throughout the day.

2. What is it like to STOP before compulsively eating?

3. Stop whatever you are doing right now. Simply press pause and take a few breaths. What is that experience like? Can you find more moments like this for yourself today?

4. Find a meditation application to download to your phone. Several exist with timers to practice stopping and finding your breath. *Headspace, Calm* and *Buddhify* are a few examples.

5. The next time you have a craving when you are not physically hungry, practice stopping. Try to delay eating for five minutes. If after five minutes you still feel you must eat, do so with awareness. Do not judge it. You still did an amazing job by just breaking up the automatic thought/behavior pattern.

6. Practice some of the breathing techniques listed above. What works for you? What can you practice so you will be ready to stop when you experience cravings but are not physically hungry?

CHAPTER 7

Observe, Isn't that Interesting?

Between the stimulus and the response there is a space. In that space is our power to choose our response. In our response lies our growth and freedom. The last of human freedoms is to choose one's attitude in any given set of circumstances.

-Viktor E. Frankl,
Austrian, psychiatrist,
survivor of Auschwitz

O is for Observe

To be successful in recovery, you must be willing to be curious. It is not enough to want to stop overeating and lose weight. Do you want to explore within? Are you willing to explore your mind? Are you willing to question your own surface reality and find your inner truths? Do you have a desire to move forward?

You may think the answer to this is obvious. Why, after all, would anyone pick up a self-help book if they were not curious about themselves? Well, they would. We often start recovery just wanting to lose weight. We have no interest in doing the hard work it takes to face the fears and emotions that fuel our disordered eating. How about you, dear reader? Are you afraid of your emotions? Do you have fears surrounding the inner drivers that fuel your disordered eating? It is okay if you are, but are you still willing to move forward?

How many of us stop and objectively observe what is going on inside of us? Mostly, I think we act on our impulses and subconscious messages without question. We respond to stressors in automatic, reactive ways. To develop new perspectives, we need to learn to step back through the "O" of SOFT AIM, "observing." What are we observing? Having learned the "S" of SOFT AIM, we have now "stopped". We stop because we recognize that something is going on. Observing will go with the next two letters of SOFT AIM, "F" for "Feeling" and "T" for "Thoughts." But for now let's just learn more about the "observer".

First and foremost, an observer is very different from a judge. An observer does not say that something is either good or bad. She is not trying to make anything happen, but just observing her immediate experience. She is interested, curious, and alert. She is simply gathering information. She is "connecting the dots." As James Baraz, co-founder of Spirit Rock Meditation Center points out, "That which is aware of fear is not itself afraid."[1] We can perceive the emotion without getting hi-jacked by the emotion. The observer allows us to objectify our emotions, and in doing so we are distanced from their effects.

Observing and understanding our thoughts is where healthy brain rewiring can take place. Just by stopping and observing, we are strengthening our prefrontal cortex. When we are observing we are present in the here and now. We are noticing our reactions. We are identifying our triggers and patterns. We are also learning to recognize that we are more than our thoughts and emotions. The part of us that is observing is indeed separate from and healthier than the part of us that usually drowns in the emotion. It is awareness and observation that combined with the rest of SOFT AIM will allow us our "Aha!" moment.

Observing also teaches us self-awareness. Self-awareness is essential to creating new options for behavior. We are learning flexibility as well. Rather than being trapped in old patterns, we are learning to respond in new and more adaptive ways. This is a great asset to have in an uncertain, ever-changing world.

Ask yourself who is the *you* that is observing? I suggest it is your healthiest self or your deeply spiritual self. This healthy part is another piece of SOFT AIM (called Mothering) that we will focus on later. It is a part of ourselves we will need to grow and develop in order to recover. It is who we really are behind our habitual patterns.

Not only is observing good for identifying the feelings and thoughts that lead us to compulsively eat, but it is a method for understanding the cycle of our disordered eating. Rather than trying to control our urge to eat, we need to get curious about how this thing works in us. Trying to control it keeps us in a tailspin.

We often think of detachment as a negative characteristic, but the "O" in SOFT AIM is best achieved through healthy detachment. Practicing healthy detachment means we accept the situation that we are in and step back to notice it. For example, we may be experiencing an uncomfortable emotion, a too long line at the grocery store, or a desire to head to the fridge when we are not hungry. Observing allows us to disengage from our unhealthy patterns and familiar traps. It allows us to see the bigger picture.

The "O" of SOFT AIM is intentionally before the "F" for feelings and the "T" for thoughts. We want to make curious contact with what we are experiencing before our thinking mind takes over. It also comes intentionally before the "M" of SOFT AIM, the mindful mothering part. We have to be a curious observer before we can recognize and utilize the last part of SOFT AIM: our healthy self-mothering voice.

Observing promotes an attitude of "Isn't that interesting?", rather than a judgment like "That's horrible or "That's frightening." Just stop and observe. What if I were to ask you to go outside and stand near the railroad tracks and tell me when a train goes by. You would say, "There it is." If you then took off running, grabbing on to the caboose and letting it drag you down the tracks, you would NOT be observing. It is the same with observing your feelings and thoughts. You need to observe, not jump on the tracks and get dragged along.

Other Benefits of Observing

In my practice, I have noticed that many of those with disordered eating are highly sensitive and very intuitive people. The word sensitive has gotten a bad rap. How many of you have been told that you are "too sensitive?" Perhaps it is all too easy for you to absorb the emotional climate around you. The "O" of SOFT AIM, can provide extra help if you are one of those acutely sensitive people. This is because when you are "observing," you are not "absorbing." Observing allows you to be supportive but not over involved.

Be aware that our craziest, most obsessive thoughts thrive on secrecy. The part of you that is healthy enough to recognize obsessing, that you are, for example, "too fat for words," does not feel talking about it would help. I agree. It would not. However, saying a code word out loud can help. Allow me to provide an example from my own life. While I don't often obsess about food or weight anymore, I do occasionally worry about things over which I have no control. Recently, while awaiting a medical test result, I could not keep from obsessing about the unknown. My thoughts were threatening to ruin the weekend. I was brooding. I told my husband what was going on and suggested the following: "Let's say I'm on a train looking out the window and my crazy thoughts about this medical test are the houses." We decided that every time I had another obsessive thought about my situation, I would just say, "house." He did not need to respond in any way to my saying "house," just hear it for me. Sometimes there were hours between the "houses." Sometimes, something would trigger me, and I would say "house, house, house!" And we would laugh. Honestly, this is what I use, and it helps a great deal. Notice, I visualized the train continuing to move. Had I stopped it and run off into any of the metaphorical houses, I would not have been observing, but rather I would have been hijacked by the emotion.

Another great way to practice the skill of observing your thoughts is through mindfulness and meditation. When I try to still my mind, I simply observe thoughts as they enter by internally saying, "Thoughts..." and returning my attention to my breath. Mindfulness also strengthens our prefrontal cortex, allows us to see more clearly, and helps us build new neural pathways.

As suggested in the last chapter on stopping, it is important to practice when the going is not so rough. Observing can be as simple as taking a moment at work between emails and busy tasks to pause and look around, noticing the sights and sounds and identifying your thoughts and feelings.

Observing means:
- You are stepping back
- You are not trying to make the situation any different than what it is.
- You are noticing life as it is happening right now.
- You are not thinking about life but experiencing it in the present.
- You are recognizing you are more than your stories about things.

Observing your feelings and thoughts is not difficult. It just involves practice. If "stop" is the hardest part, "observing" might be the most important. When you are observing, you are aware that you are NOT your thoughts or your feelings.

The mind will not be happy about observing. It will try to distract you and put you back under its spell. Remember, do not judge your feelings or thoughts even as you figure out how silly most of them are. Just recognize that they are fabrications of a mind that believes it must control and resist everything to be safe. The irony is that the more you try to control life, the more out of control it becomes. The more you can stop and get curious about observing what is happening, right now, the happier you will be. You are moving out of struggle and resistance and into living more fully.

Practice Observing Thoughts

Find a comfortable place where you will not be disturbed. Sit or lie in a comfortable position. Attempt to slow your mind. This is usually best achieved by focusing on the slow rhythmic in and out of your breath. Simply observe when your thoughts enter. Notice the gaps between your thoughts. When the thoughts enter, gently let them go by returning to your breath.

Whenever you become aware that you are lost in your thoughts, back up and return to observing. Try out some of the following visualization exercises.

- Imagine yourself sitting at the edge of a riverbank. See your thoughts like leaves, floating by on the surface of the water
- Ducks have a protective coating which allows rain to roll off their backs. Imagine your thoughts are like beads of rain rolling off into the water.
- Imagine your thoughts as clouds floating by.
- Imagine your thoughts as planes or birds going by.
- Imagine your thoughts as the aforementioned train disappearing over the horizon.
- Imagine yourself sitting in a train, enjoying the countryside rolling by. Your thoughts are the houses. They appear and are gone. You can imagine yourself saying "house" each time you have a thought. And poof, the houses disappear as the train keeps moving.

What is coming up for you right now? Are you an observer of your responses or are you merely reacting to life's circumstances?

Practice observing. Set the intention that you will start being more observant and therefore more self-aware. At random times, notice how you feel in your body, how you feel emotionally and mentally. Observe non-judgmentally.

CHAPTER 8

F is for Feeling

The reason we suffer from our emotion is not because of emotion itself, but because of our resistance to that particular
-Teal Swan

By now, you are working on:
1. Improving your self-talk.
2. Recognizing and eating from physical hunger.
3. Matching hunger to what your body wants.
4. Learning when to stop eating by identifying satiety.
5. Leaning into recovery in a gentler way through SOFT AIM.
6. Stopping whenever you want to eat and are not hungry.
7. Observing what is happening at the moment you want to eat but are not hungry.

This chapter is about learning to recognize and observe our feelings. Most of us have a great deal to learn about emotions, also known as feelings. First and foremost, feelings are messengers. They tell us that something needs to be paid attention to. Maybe we are feeling anger. Perhaps anger is paying us a visit because it wants us to recognize that a boundary is being violated or an injustice is being committed. Maybe sadness has swept in because we need to heal or release old hurts. Maybe we just need to have a good cry. For males and females, crying is the appropriate response to sadness. An emotion we like to squelch is fear. As we learned about in an earlier chapter, fear is a legacy from our ancestors. It is hardwired. Anxiety helped them survive. The individual who was not concerned about becoming prey, likely did, and thus, died. Now, however, we over-react to situations. We respond as if there is a saber tooth tiger at our door when, in reality, it is only UPS.

The point is, we must face our emotions. If we don't, they will keep us stuck. Only by facing our difficult emotions can we find the courage to transform them. All too often, we are embarrassed and ashamed, desperate to stuff those nasty feelings down with food. But SOFT AIM's "observing" way of recognizing our emotions makes them more manageable.

Regardless of the emotion, recovery demands we change to an "equal opportunity" policy with our feelings. It does not demand we like them all the same, but we have to accept that none are good or bad or right or wrong. Emotions just are. We must change our attitude from avoidance and judgment to curiosity and compassion.

Emotions are energy. And energy can be blocked, or it can flow. When we use our disordered relationship with food, weight and body to ignore our feelings, we are blocking that energy. Unfortunately, the energy is still there. It is just stuck. Emotions that have been stuffed down and stuck manifest in unhealthy and increasingly dysfunctional ways.

So, here is both the hard and easy part. Every time you have the desire for food and you are not hungry, acknowledge that something is wrong. Your job is to figure it out. Okay, maybe not EVERY time as even "normal eaters" might want that extra piece of pecan pie at Grandma's house on Thanksgiving. Let's just say that most of the time when you eat, physical hunger--not an emotion--should be the cue. This means you have a lot of work to do. On the bright side, your dis-ordered eating provides you a sure fire way to recognize if something in you is in need of attention.

Jane Hirshmann and Carol H. Munter in their book "Overcoming

Overeating" said that overeaters have a "calming" problem, not an "eating" problem.[1] Food is the tool overeaters use to calm themselves from difficult emotions. For some, nearly every emotion gives discomfort.

Why do we feed our emotions? The reasons are complex. Let's start with gender roles and our culture. A very interesting study, conducted by Inge Broverman, illustrates one of the reasons we have numbed ourselves from emotions.[2] This study set out to determine how sex influenced a clinician's definition of a psychologically healthy adult.

Broverman asked 79 mental health professionals to use a stereotype questionnaire to describe a mature, healthy adult. Some of the participants were asked only to describe a male, others a female, and the rest were asked to describe a healthy adult with an unspecified gender. The results indicated that participants believed that a healthy adult and a healthy male shared virtually all the same characteristics. A healthy female, however, was thought to possess different qualities.

Adults and males were said to share a "competence cluster" of traits such as confidence and independence. Women, on the other hand, had a "warmth-expressiveness cluster" that described kindness and concern for others. These results put women in a no-win situation. If they demonstrated the traits considered healthy for a female, they were simultaneously classified as an unhealthy, psychologically immature adult. But if they demonstrated the traits of a healthy adult, they were classified as an unhealthy female. In essence, women are damned if they do, and damned if they don't.

Our family of origin often plays a role in how we have come to use food to handle our emotions. Perhaps you were a sensitive child. Maybe you were scolded for crying too often or even called a "baby." Perhaps you heard the particularly horrible, "I'll give you something to cry about." Maybe your parents or others in your family did not value the expression of feelings in themselves or in you. Perhaps you received such a poor example of expression of feelings that you decided to keep your feelings to yourself. Maybe expression of feelings was simply not safe. Regardless of the reason or reasons, you likely have much to learn about emotions.

More evidence for the need to recognize and accept our emotions comes from the groundbreaking book by Daniel Goleman, entitled, *Emotional Intelligence*. Goleman says:

> Emotions streamline our decisions at the outset by eliminating some options and highlighting others. Emotions guide us in facing predicaments and tasks too important to leave to intellect alone: danger, painful loss, persisting toward a goal despite frustrations, bonding with a mate and building a family. When it comes to shaping our most important decisions and actions, the emotional brain is as involved in reasoning as the thinking brain.[3]

Another issue with denying our emotions is that we do not get to "selectively numb." The degree to which we numb those uncomfortable emotions, is the same degree to which we fail to experience feelings of joy and happiness. Everything becomes blunted.

Denying our emotions does not work. Eating our way through sadness or anger only makes us numb. It does nothing to solve our emotional issues. If you eat because you are depressed, you are even more depressed after the "binge numb" wears off. The same happens if you eat because of anxiety or loneliness and so on.

We can learn a great deal from the addictions model of recovery. Several behaviors have been shown to predict relapse, most notably avoidance behaviors. When an addict is gearing up for a relapse he or she tries to avoid pain and is often anxious and angry. This, of course, releases adrenaline and speeds up the body. It depletes endorphins (feel good chemical) and ends with exhaustion. And then, feeling hopeless, the addict succumbs to use again.

I hope you are gaining insight into your patterns of emotional expression. Perhaps you ask why you should bother with all these uncomfortable feelings? Isn't it easier to just stuff them down? To that I state a resounding "NO!" Emotional eating comes at a cost. I am not talking about the cost of excess weight or obesity related diseases. I am not talking about your self-esteem being affected by your jean size or about failing to lose that 30 pounds for your niece's wedding.

I am talking about "soul" loss. I am talking about being stuck living a half-life. As long as you are using and abusing food, you don't have to leave a disappointing relationship, quit a miserable job, take a dream trip, or take up a new hobby. Instead, you focus on drowning in the next binge or alternately losing that weight once and for all. Then, at goal weight, your life can finally begin. In the meantime, life piles up. Stuffed emotions pile up and surface in often horrid ways. One way those years of buried emotions come out is in your physical health. But even health scares don't motivate change because the prescription for change is yet another diet. And that never really works. Climbing out of this pattern sounds daunting and because we don't know where to start, we don't. And the years roll on.

I suspect that the idea of recognizing emotions and changing your relationship to them sounds difficult. Remember, we live in an emotionally illiterate society; we may well have been raised to ignore our emotions. Working through emotions INSTEAD of binging probably sounds next to impossible.

Time to remind you that recovery is a non-linear process. That means it is a jumbled up, long-term deal and not an easy fix. Food will continue to be a necessary part of your life. Indeed, hunger is a sign of your good health. Losing one's appetite is often a sign of disease.

So, where is a good place to start? Something I did in my own recovery that helped me and took very little time was to randomly check in with myself several times a day to go over various emotions and rate them. I would usually write on a piece of scratch paper the following: H for happy, S for sad, A for angry, AN for anxious. Then I would rate each emotion on a 1 to 10 scale with 10 being the most intense and 1 the least. I wanted to see in which emotional landscape I dwelled. And I learned. I learned a lot. I learned that happiness and joy were all too infrequent visitors. I learned that my primary dominant emotion was anxiety. I did not like finding out that I lived with so much fear. But it did help me develop that compassion for myself. It also helped me learn to OBSERVE and tolerate difficult emotions. Even if it was only for a few moments before I defaulted to an old behavior, I was developing emotional tolerance.

Many of us have no idea what we are feeling or that each feeling manifests somewhere in our body. We confuse feelings with thoughts. We also think that if we do recognize a feeling, the thoughts that created it must be true. In fact, it is our old neural wiring that has run amuck, leaving us breathless and eating our way through life. If you don't want to spend the rest of your life throwing cookies at every problem, you need to learn the difference between thoughts and emotions. The next chapter will make that difference clear.

Journal Assignment
**Remember when working on identifying feelings to do so in the observing way we learned about in the last chapter.

1. What did you learn about feelings from your family of origin? From your mother, your father, or anyone else?
2. How do you think culture and the media have influenced the way you process emotions?
3. Take a moment to rate yourself on each of the following emotions. On a 1-10 scale with ten being the highest, where are you in terms of joy, sadness, anger, fear? Check and recheck. See if you can learn to recognize emotions easier and when you are stuck in any particular emotion.
4. Try to locate the emotion you identified in #3 in your body. If you cannot identify an emotion in #3, start with your body. Are your shoulders tight? What emotion might that be about?
5. What do you think about the first three letters of SOFT AIM; *stopping* and *observing* your *feelings*?

CHAPTER 9

T is for Thoughts

The mind is a wonderful servant but a terrible master.
-Robin S. Sharma

The T in SOFT AIM is for thought. As you learned in the previous chapter, every feeling is a messenger. And the message can be found in the thought. For example, if you feel sadness, there is a thought that is producing sadness. If you feel angry, there is a thought that tells you that a wrong has been committed.

I use the following exercise with my clients to illustrate how their thoughts about and perception of an event determine their emotional response.

There is a high school. The fire alarm goes off. There is an event, a thought, and a resulting feeling.

Girl #1
Event: fire alarm sounds
Thought: "Oh no. The building is on fire!"
Feeling: Fear and panic

Girl #2
Event: fire alarm sounds

THE HANDS THAT FEED ME

Thought: "Oh great. I just washed my hair and now we have to go outside in the rain where it will be ruined."
Feeling: Annoyed

Girl#3
Event: fire alarm sounds
Thought: "Yay! The fire alarm is sounding so we won't have to take that quiz today after all!"
Feeling: Relief, happiness

As you can see in this example, the same event produced a variety of responses depending on how it was perceived by each student. It was the thoughts *about* the event, not the event itself, which led to the experienced emotion.

This might be okay if minds weren't such elaborate "storytellers". It is the mind's task to constantly analyze and interpret events in our outer world. The way the mind interprets events is based on our past experiences and own unique wiring. You may have themes and even favorite genres to your inner rantings. Perhaps you are always the victim or maybe the persecutor. Maybe your genre is horror or suspense.

Whatever your theme or genre, your thoughts are something you usually do not question. Robert Burton, a neurologist, says that our brains reward us with dopamine when we recognize and complete patterns.[1] Your repetitive thoughts, or stories as Burton calls them, are recognized as patterns. These stories do not have to be true and are often based on past patterns of dysfunction that you may have learned at a younger age.

I once had a client who spent most of an hour upset because she was sure her husband and children were going to forget her birthday. She noted they had barely mentioned it, and apparently everyone already had other plans on her birthday weekend. This story went with her ongoing theme that she was taken for granted and often forgotten. At the next session, she sheepishly admitted that the reason everything had been so quiet was that they had planned an elaborate surprise party for her.

In spite of reality checks like the one above, it will still be difficult to remember that thoughts are just thoughts and not necessarily true. The mind talks incessantly and unfortunately it is more interested in controlling life than experiencing it. It will not like you objectively observing your feelings and thoughts. It will fight it. Like an addict, it wants its shot of dopamine. It will insist you are right in whatever your story is.

Teasing out the thoughts and emotions/feelings leading to the binge/restrict cycle is a challenging task. This is because you are trying to make the unconscious, conscious. Changing neural patterns takes intense awareness. You are becoming aware of your thoughts in an "observing" curious way. You are meeting yourself where you are before you try to change anything.

Core Beliefs

Related to thoughts are core beliefs. Core beliefs describe the very essence of how you see yourself, others, and the world around you. They have been learned, rehearsed, and shaped to form your self-perception. They are, by nature, inflexible and deeply ingrained. Unfortunately, many of your core beliefs are likely MISPERCEPTIONS which can sound something like this: "I am incompetent; I am untrustworthy, good things never happen to me." To complicate matters, they operate beneath your consciousness and their validity is seldom questioned. Rather, you strive to maintain them and go so far as to create stories and compile evidence to affirm them. These core beliefs become ingrained into your neural network. They produce involuntary and often illogical thoughts which come to mind when a particular situation occurs. Let's say, for example, you have a core belief in your incompetence. You will unconsciously create situations to prove you are correct in this assumption. Indeed your brain delights in supplying evidence for your core beliefs.

Triggers

A trigger is something that elicits a conditioned response that pushes you toward the binge/restrict cycle. We all have personal triggers. For example, a trigger for a person with disordered eating could include any of the following:

- An argument with your mother, father, child, sibling or spouse
- A comment about your weight, body, or food choices
- Someone talking about a certain food that you then crave and decide to binge on
- A bad grade on a test or assignment
- Getting reprimanded at work
- Being at an event and having social anxiety
- Alcohol and substance use
- Hormones
- The season
- Tight or uncomfortable clothing
- Scale
- Money

One of your goals is to get to know your triggers. Becoming aware what situations set off the binge/restrict cycle will help you to head them off.

Vulnerabilities

Vulnerabilities are those personal traits that make you more susceptible to triggers and to the binge/restrict cycle. Vulnerabilities are different for different people. You need to learn yours. The following are typical vulnerabilities:

- Being tired
- Letting yourself get too hungry
- Physical pain
- Being emotionally worn out

- Fears related to scarcity such as not enough money, clothes, food etc.
- The feeling that you are not enough
- Poor self-care
- Too much structure and/or busyness
- Too little structure, chaos
- Too much down time and/or boredom

You need to be able to identify both your triggers and your vulnerabilities. You must do your best to avoid or at least anticipate them.

Where to Start

Initially, you may only be able to recognize the feelings present AFTER a binge. While the feelings when you restrict are usually a mix of guilt (depending on your level of deprivation) and a sense of control, the feelings post binge are usually ambivalence, numbness, and shame.

Eventually, you will recognize the binge while in the binge. I often have clients tell me that I have ruined binging for them because they can no longer stay unconscious. They may be binging, but they are very aware of what they are feeling or trying not to feel and why. The goal is to be aware and stop before the binge. This will require you to be patient with yourself.

The first task is to recognize how emotions and accompanying thoughts connect to your disordered eating. This requires focused attention and detective work. You need to recognize that when you want to eat and you are not hungry, something is amiss. It is time to figure out what that is.

The Science

Hopefully, you are starting to understand that binges are not simply mindless and meaningless experiences. They are mindless, only when you are in them. The buildup to the binge is very specific and full of information and clues. To stop the binging pattern you have to make the unconscious thoughts and patterns conscious.

To complicate matters, researchers have shown that the brains of overeaters may have an abnormality in the way endorphins are metabolized. These findings are in line with theories that say overeating, like other addictions, is partly due to a problem in the reward center of the brain. Compulsive overeaters may have an over dependence on rewards which is thought to be connected to the hypothalamus.[2] They may actually be eating because they need more serotonin. In addition, they likely have trouble regulating their emotions. Back to that overly developed amygdala that sees danger everywhere. If you have had any trauma, it is safe to say your amygdala may be in overdrive. Slowing down the compulsive process takes deliberate awareness.

When you have a repetitive thought, your brain helps by wiring the thought in so fully that you are not even aware you are having it. You are only conscious of your thinking when it is a new thought. The rest is too fast to recognize. And the only way to figure that out is through the "F" or "feeling" part of SOFT AIM.

As you learned in the previous chapter, you must find the feeling, then identify the accompanying thought. This is important as your thoughts shape your life. When you are not aware of our thoughts, they rule you. As the quote at the beginning of this chapter says, you want your mind (thoughts) to be servant to your highest good, not the master. You have to become aware of your thoughts before you can gain any mastery over them.

The Good News

The good news is that thoughts can change. When you change your thinking, you can regulate your emotions and improve your life. Physiologically, emotions only last for about a minute. It is your thoughts that can keep them in a perpetual, never-ending loop.[3] In addition, you often don't realize how your core beliefs hold you back in life. While it will likely be challenging to unearth and change your thoughts and beliefs, the more you do this, the more room you create for a better more fulfilling life. Are you starting to see how just going on a diet does not really fix anything? Can you forgive yourself for all the pounds lost and regained? Until you change your thoughts through SOFT AIM, the weight loss will likely not stick, and you will be stuck in the perpetual cycle of restriction and binging.

Putting our Thoughts in Second Person

As previously mentioned in Chapter 2, a technique I have used with clients is to put thoughts into second person. For example, when you recognize the feeling, say, "Hello fear. What do you have to say today?" And from there, let the story pour forth.

For me, fear is usually like my six year old self. "But what if?" She stammers on and on, creating elaborate catastrophes. Anger is a little older and usually pretty rebellious and defensive. This second person technique will also help when it is time to access the M of SOFT AIM, the Mindful-Mothering piece.

You may feel a sense of apprehension about identifying your feelings and thoughts, but you don't need to fear them. Simply listen and be curious. They are usually not as unmanageable as you think. They are like the shadow on the wall that looks like a monster to a child. When you *stop* to recognize your *feelings* and *thoughts* in the *observing* way of SOFT AIM, you are turning the light on in that dark room. You realize the monster is just the shadow of a stuffed toy on the chair.

Journal Assignment

1. Practice the SOFT of SOFT AIM. Stop and observe. What is the feeling that you are experiencing right now? What is the thought behind the feeling? Write it down. Practice doing this regularly. You are checking in with yourself in a new way.

2. What are some of your triggers? How about your vulnerabilities? How do they play into your emotional eating? What can you do differently to prepare for or avoid your triggers and vulnerabilities?

3. Practice directly addressing your thoughts. Use second person to acknowledge and challenge those automatic, involuntary thoughts which trigger binge-eating.

CHAPTER 10

A is for Allow

The Guest House
This being human is a guest house.
Every morning a new arrival.

A joy, a depression, a meanness,
some momentary awareness comes
as an unexpected visitor.

Welcome and entertain them all!
Even if they're a crowd of sorrows,
who violently sweep your house
empty of its furniture,
still treat each guest honorably.
He may be clearing you out
for some new delight.

The dark thought, the shame, the malice,
meet them at the door laughing,
and invite them in.

Be grateful for whoever comes,
because each has been sent
as a guide from beyond.

-Rumi

I love this poem by Rumi. It captures the true art of "allowing" which is an important part of the practice of SOFT AIM. For in SOFT AIM, we are not fighting or resisting. We are meeting life "at the door". "Welcoming" as Rumi writes. Rumi reminds us to be grateful, for even our difficult emotions because "each has been sent as a guide from beyond."

Now, not only are you stopping and observing your feelings and thoughts, you are allowing them. It is in NOT allowing that you rush to numb yourself through binging and restricting. If your feeling is "sadness", you can say, "Hello sadness. There you are." If your thoughts are catastrophic and hopeless, you still need to meet them where they are.

If you are embracing the "O" of SOFT AIM and non-judgmentally observing, then the "A" for allowing will be much easier. Since you are detaching yourself from how you think things should be, without the filter of judgment, you can experience the truth of the present moment. You can simply allow for things to be as they are. As hard as this may sound, observing combined with allowing will bring you peace. Where has not allowing ever got you? It is like standing in a rain storm cursing at the sky. Good for you. Curse away. Guess what? It is still raining. As author and teacher Byron Katie says, "When you argue with reality, you lose, but only 100% of the time."[1]

Sadly, you really are not in control of your life nearly as much as you think you are. But that is okay. You do not have to be afraid. I don't claim to understand why children starve and genocides happen, but I still choose to believe we live in a purposeful universe. By this I mean we can trust that we do not have to be in charge. You can lean into adversity instead of stuffing it down with food. You can even shift your focus to one of believing that even the tough things in life offer the possibility of blessings and growth. Mary O'Malley, author of what's in the way is the way, suggests we move from a "life is happening TO me" paradigm to a "life is happening FOR me."[2] Put simply, she suggests life struggles are there for us to learn from.

Ironically, the more you try to control your food compulsions, the more you lose. It is only in SOFT AIM and through gentle observing and allowing that the compulsion loosens its grip.

Remember, you don't have to like or agree with something to allow it. This is NOT "positive thinking." It is very different from that. Positive thinking is what you may try in an attempt to escape from discomfort, but it doesn't work. Being optimistic is great, but it is not enough. Emotions are simply *energy in motion*. They need to move through your body. They are neither good nor bad. They need only to be experienced. And they are directly connected to your thoughts.

The practice of allowing will cultivate the work of acceptance. Marsha Linehan, the psychologist who created Dialectical Behavioral Therapy, more commonly known as DBT,[3] and Tara Brach, a meditation teacher and author, both talk about "radical acceptance"[4] which suggests that we accept the reality of what is in this moment. It means choosing to not resist what can't be changed. It is about saying yes to life, just as it is.

To use the oft quoted recovery slogan: "Accept life on life's terms." Say yes to what you have no real control over. In the case of the A of SOFT AIM, it means allowing the moment that is here. Allowing it without judgment, even if it is illogical, irrational or a bit scary.

Yes, allowing is often difficult. It can be downright painful. It is, however, emotionally detrimental to push experiences away and fight reality. Not allowing equates with continued suffering. To avoid suffering, you are likely to engage in a disordered relationship with food.

Exercise provides us with a good metaphor for this situation. When you start an exercise program, if you are pushing yourself at all, you will experience muscle soreness. But the soreness indicates that you are getting stronger. It tells you that you are working hard and getting stronger. Allowing your feelings and thoughts is no different. You will feel pain, but like the pain of exercise, you are becoming stronger.

Part of the reason allowing is so hard is that we tend to think that by fighting reality we are not "giving in". We believe we will ultimately win and control life. Although, that may be true for some things, it is not the case here. Unpredictable things happen in every life. Allowing takes practice.

Begin practicing allowing with little things like a missed phone call, a too long red light, or a lost parking spot. Focus on your breath. Observe the thoughts that you have about the situation. Then practice acceptance. You may try saying softly, "It is what it is." Breathe and practice letting it go with your exhale. Let yourself feel the peace of allowing. When you allow, you open up the space for positive change to actually happen. Ironically, you may be more likely to lose weight when you stop obsessing about weight loss and allow your experiences.

Allowing helps your brain become more resilient. You cultivate inner strength. In addition it grounds you in the here and now. This is where life is actually happening. This is the **only** place life is happening. Since you will no longer be dominated by fear and avoidance, you can become yourself. You may wonder who you actually are underneath the fear and avoidance. One way to find that true self is to become very clear on your values. What are the values that you hold most dear? My top two are compassion and perseverance. So, when I am looking for my "true north", it is these values that guide me, not my fearful self.

Allowing is more than just a letter of SOFT AIM; it is also part of the overall approach. When you don't allow, you constrict or tense up, making whatever you are feeling more intense. You revert to the stress response. When you are in the stress response, you are, among other things, over-producing cortisol which contributes to weight gain and obesity. Allowing puts you into the creative flow of recovery. You acknowledge you are seeking a recovery but you are aiming softly, without force or tension.

Interestingly, the physical and emotional body works similarly. If you have ever dealt with physical pain, you may have been told to "breathe into it." That is because tensing up constricts the area and makes the pain worse. Have you ever had a headache? If you are paying attention, you will become aware of how resisting it makes the pain worse. It works the same with recovery. You need to lean into and breathe into both physical and emotional pain. Your goal is not to make pain magically disappear but to reduce your suffering. As the famous line goes, "resistance is futile."

Make no mistake, this is no small feat. You are overriding your automatic fight/flight response. Not only that, but you are allowing life to pass through you. It means no more resisting or controlling. You may, after some practice, actually come to trust that life is working for you. Even when you don't like it, you can learn to trust it. You may after casting a gentle light on the stories of your life, be able to let them go. You may come up with new ways to navigate your world and your food. Life becomes more than a series of random and sometimes threatening events you need to guard against or outmaneuver. Allowing means you are no longer the victim.

The last line in the Rumi poem talks about each guest (feeling) being sent like a guide from beyond. What a great reminder that there is a message in your suffering that you can hear, if you are willing to listen and allow. Only in fully allowing and honoring your feelings will you be able to move to the next parts of SOFT AIM, the practice of Investigation and self-*Mothering*. In these steps, you are going to allow your intuition to investigate the thought and help you work through whatever is going on.

In summary, allowing is **not**:
- manipulating
- controlling
- judging
- fixing
- positive thinking
- necessarily agreeing
- passivity

Allowing is:
- trusting

- being patient
- having faith
- letting feelings be what they are
- being courageous
- liberating

Practice

Practice allowing. Practice viewing your emotional pain as an opportunity for growth. You can do this daily through prayer, meditation or simply putting your attention and awareness on allowing things to be as they are. Have faith that they will work out. Talk about this with a friend. Ask for support as you learn to fight less and allow more.

Journal Assignment

1. Reflect on the statement: "Our challenge is to allow life to pass through us instead of making it a certain way."
2. What feelings and thoughts does that statement bring up for you? Allow them. Do you feel any resistance to allowing your experience to be what it is?
3. Do you allow yourself to experience your feelings? Why or why not? If not, how would allowing yourself to feel a full range of emotions, transform your recovery and life?
4. Are you willing to endure the discomfort of allowing? Are you willing to push your limits in order to get stronger?

CHAPTER 11

Investigate Like CSI

> Thoughts believed create your world. When you question
> your thoughts, you change your world.
>
> *Byron Katie*

Our brains are amazing. Through repetition, we establish patterns of behavior, learn conditioned responses, and develop habits. Unfortunately, some of those patterns, responses and habits can become physically and psychologically damaging. Disordered eating, for example, begins with an unconscious automatic (habitual) response to a particular situation (or emotional trigger). To achieve recovery, we must break down the old patterns and build new neural pathways in our brain. To do so, we must first become aware of the old pathways through the STOP, OBSERVE, FEELING, THOUGHT and ALLOW parts of SOFT AIM. Then, through INVESTIGATION, we can begin constructing new and improved pathways through conscious focus and intent. When we investigate our current, often dysfunctional story, we light up the neural network, making it available for rewiring. If we are not observing the thought, we are imbedded in it. And no change happens. Actually, we may even strengthen the unhealthy thought if we are not in a detached observing mode.

In this chapter we are going to explore the "I" of SOFT AIM: *Investigate*. This is where we start to tease apart our story and let our healthy self-mothering voice assist in balancing our thoughts.

Our stories often come from a younger frightened part of our psyche. They are the culmination of every trauma or slight we have ever endured. Investigation requires rigorous honesty. It also requires daring. We, in effect, are questioning the truth of our reality because the story we tell about our situation does indeed feel like reality. It is also about questioning authority. What authority you may ask? You! Your own mind and every unquestioned assumption. In addition you are investigating your thoughts as if they are a crime scene. That means objectively, without judgment. Back to that interested observer.

One of my favorite proponents of questioning your thoughts is the famous writer and speaker, Byron Katie. I highly recommend Katie's first book, *Loving What Is*.[1] Katie teaches a process she calls, "The Work." The basis of the work is a series of four questions addressed to your own lists of written assumptions. Whether you're angry with your spouse, frustrated with your teen, or appalled by the state of the world, Katie suggests you write down your honest thoughts on the matter. Then, begin the examination. Start with, "Is it true?" and continue exploring of "Who would I be without that thought?"

Another impressive aspect of the process is called, "the turnaround." This is where you turn around every problem you have with anyone or anything else on yourself. If you decide that your spouse is selfish, the turnaround forces you to examine ways that you are selfish.

One of the things I like about The Work is that Katie encourages us to WRITE down our thoughts and judgments. As always, and with all of SOFT AIM, your process will be enhanced if you write it down. Sometimes, just the act of writing things down will help you to see the errors in your thinking.

It is important to investigate your thoughts and stories because your stories, which are often worst case scenarios and victim thinking, keep you anxious and depressed. Depression and anxiety hinder healing. Psychotropic medication can only go so far. It is up to you to change your thinking; and that is what the "I" of SOFT AIM is about. Your mind may be caught in such a negative spiral that more balanced thinking will be very difficult. You may even think that you do not deserve to be happy or peaceful. Back to the core beliefs we learned about in the chapter on thoughts. Every thought we have releases chemicals in the brain. Peaceful and hopeful thoughts release chemicals that help us feel hopeful and calm. Negative thoughts release chemicals that make us feel anxious and sad.

Cognitive behavioral therapy has identified some typical thought patterns that affect compulsive eaters. When you investigate your thoughts, you are engaging in the process of cognitive restructuring. You are replacing worn out, outdated modes of thinking with more helpful ones. Although there are more thought patterns than what are listed here, these are the ones that frequently affect those with disordered eating.

- **Catastrophizing.** Seeing only the worst possible outcome in everything. For example, you ate a dessert, so now you will gain 100 pounds. Alternately, this could be in the form of making one small mistake and deciding you are hopeless. Remember the internal "critic" we talked about in Chapter 2? She is quite adept with catastrophizing.
- **Minimization and magnification.** On one hand we catastrophize our disordered eating; on the other hand we minimize its effect. Example: "This binge does not matter. I will start again tomorrow or Monday or after the holidays." Overeaters tend to do magnification in the literal sense. They usually have a distorted body image, seeing themselves as much larger than they actually are. This may be the "hell with it" voice we talked about in Chapter 2. The one who said finishing off the pie was not a big deal.
- **Leaps in logic.** Making seemingly logic-based statements, even though there is no real evidence to support them. You jump to conclusions, usually negative ones. One type of illogical leap is assuming that you know what someone else is

thinking. Size discrimination is alive and well, but if you are a compulsive eater who is also very overweight, you may blame your size on everything. For example: "They did not pick me for the promotion because I am fat." "They are looking at me and thinking I am so big and fat." Another leap of logic you may make is that you are a failure for every binge, diet failure or every pound gained or not lost.

- **"All or nothing" thinking.** Being unable to see shades of gray in everyday life can lead to major misperceptions and even despair. A person who thinks only in black-and-white terms can't comprehend small successes. You are either following your diet or "blowing it." You have good days and bad days, but nothing in between. This one is very problematic because recovery is neither black nor white. It is many shades of gray. Eating past fullness at one meal, just means you may need to wait a little longer until you are hungry for the next eating experience.
- **Emotional reasoning.** This error in thinking involves all of our unquestioned thoughts. We do not understand that just because we think we are stupid, does not make it so. When we engage in emotional reasoning rather than logical reasoning, we assume something is true just because we think it.

There are other irrational thoughts that left uninvestigated can lead to overeating. To name but a few: needing others' approval, general worries, social anxiety, perceiving you are being attacked if others don't agree with you, and not forgiving your own mistakes. A signal that you may be on the irrational track is when you hear yourself saying words like: never, no one, always, only and every.

You are going to learn to use your mothering voice (the "M" of SOFT AIM) in the next chapter to change your thinking. But how do you begin the INVESTIGATION? You start by asking yourself questions: Is there any evidence to support the truth of my thought? Does this thought help my recovery and mental health? Does this thought lead to self-defeating behavior? Does this thought promote problem solving? Would I offer this thought to someone else who was struggling? How do I feel when I think this thought? Remember, investigation has to be conscious and requires both time and effort.

Another way of knowing that your thought needs investigating is to put it up against your core values. For example, one of my core values is compassion. I really try to apply it everywhere. I was surprised to realize that I am not being very compassionate with myself when I overload my schedule, refuse to ask for help, or put everyone else's needs ahead of my own. Do I want to be congruent? Do I want to be authentic? Then I must make sure my core value of compassion applies to me as well as others. Core values are positive attributes such as: caring, strength, perseverance, courage, assertiveness, justice, mercy, trust, loyalty, friendliness, commitment and integrity. To be congruent your core values need to apply in your relationship with yourself. A good place to start is by identifying and investigating your thoughts.

The "I" of SOFT AIM is going to be utilized with the "M" for Mothering in the next chapter. This is not about turning every negative into a positive. Truth is, if you are a weaver of doom and gloom stories, your using stories to protect yourself from disappointment. You can lean into replacing your thoughts with more balanced ones. For example, if you are having a bad day, your internal monologue might go something like, "I hate my life. It sucks." You do not have to change it to, "Life is great!" Easing in could take the form of a response like, "Everyone has rough days. That is life."

Investigating your thoughts means you are recognizing many of your worst fears. You have to face your fears from a safe place and SOFT AIM allows you to do that. It gives you the calm you need to sort out the mess.

There is an old Cherokee tale about two wolves that can help you understand the importance of investigation:

One evening an old Cherokee Indian told his grandson about a battle that goes on inside people. He said, "My son, the battle is between two wolves inside us all. One is Evil. It is anger, envy, jealousy, sorrow, regret, greed, arrogance, self-pity, guilt, resentment, inferiority, lies, false pride, superiority, and ego. The other is good. It is joy, peace, love, hope, serenity, humility, kindness, benevolence, empathy, generosity, truth, compassion, and faith."

The grandson thought about it for a minute and then asked his grandfather, "Which wolf wins?"

The old man simply replied, "The one you feed."

How about you, dear reader? Who are you feeding? We all have a good and an evil wolf. They are fed daily by the choices we make with our thoughts. What you think about and dwell upon will, in a sense, appear in your life and influence your behavior.

You have a choice. Feed the Good Wolf and it will show up in your character, habits and life choices. Or feed the Evil Wolf and your whole world stays in anxiety and depression. The bad wolf feeds off your reactions. When you accept your thoughts without question, you feed them. If you can stop feeding your wolf, it will get weaker and weaker and eventually move on. Others will come, but again you can choose not to feed the evil wolf. You can change the way you think and react by paying more attention to the Good Wolf in you. The Good Wolf is activated when you use the last part of SOFT AIM. This strategy, called Mothering, will be covered in depth in the next chapter. The crucial question for you is "Which wolf are you feeding today?"

Journal Assignment

1. Which wolf are you feeding? Is your mind the master or the servant? Are you able to discern the truth, or do you ride on the wind of whatever the running storyline of the day is? Identify what part of your recurrent stories (thoughts) might be part of your old negative core beliefs or thought patterns.

2. What do you think might be the payoff for your negative thought patterns? Is there part of you that believes that they keep you safe?

3. How are you doing at recognizing thoughts that need to be investigated?
4. What irrational beliefs does your mind engage in?
5. What are your core values? Are you living in congruence with them?
6. How would investigating your thoughts influence your recovery?
7. Are you willing to let go of your stories?

CHAPTER 12

M is for Mother

I am larger and better than I thought. I did not know I held so much goodness.

-Walt Whitman

As we learned in the last chapter, when we investigate the stories of our mind, we will find they are often versions of a younger scared self. This part of ourselves is usually psychologically immature and irrational. It is overly concerned with safety and security. It reacts unconsciously from past traumas. These traumas can be old childhood incidents or recent losses and disappointments. Our reactions can come from societal influences and our desire for approval.

A few years ago, I fell victim to a telephone scam. A company contacted me and the caller asked a few simple questions to which I answered yes. Then my voice, saying yes, was spliced agreeing to buy a $500 subscription. They were threatening to sue me and harassing me for the money. On one occasion, I remember a particularly nasty conversation with them in which I refused to give them any money. I slammed down the phone and started pacing the house. Some years earlier, I would have found myself knee deep in snack foods, but fortunately, I was far into recovery by then.

After a few minutes, I remembered that I should practice what I preach. I sat down. I stopped. I observed what I was feeling and I saw it was high anxiety. I began investigating my thoughts. I could clearly feel my scared little six year old self. "What's the matter sweetheart?" I asked from my healthy mothering self. She stammered, "You better just pay them. What if they really sue you and ruin your credit? You need to buy a car soon and that would be terrible. Maybe they will make you go to court! They are based in New York! What if they make you fly to New York for this? What if there are court costs and lawyer fees. You really messed up by talking to them at all. You should have known it was a scam. If you were a better business person you would have. Just pay up and be done with this. Lesson learned."

At this point self-mothering kicked in. "No, you are not going to pay it. If you let them get away with this, more people will be hurt. But you are right. Their harassment is a problem. Contact the Better Business Bureau and the Attorney General's Office. It might be worth a little money to get your attorney to write a threatening letter to them as well." Done.

By moving to the mother voice and not letting my life be led by my scared six year old self, I was able to actually problem solve. This plan made me feel safe; I had the situation under control. And it worked. After my attorney's letter and a letter from the Attorney General's office, the scammers sent me a "sorry-for-the- misunderstanding" letter. My fear, my younger self, would have had me violate my principles of fairness and helping others. My true self was strong enough to stand up for what was right and not pay them. My scared younger self would have caved under pressure. As you can see from this example, it was important to allow the fearful part of myself to speak up while I was investigating.

By recognizing that the stories we are investigating usually come from a frightened child, we can understand why it is the mother voice that needs to restore us to sanity. This frightened part will just fight harder and get emotionally sicker if it feels unaccepted or unheard. We have to understand and soothe our frightened self. She needs to trust that the healthiest self is behind the steering wheel.

A good mother is neither overly permissive nor overly authoritarian.

She does not ridicule nor does she tell you to drown your sorrows in a bowl of ice cream. Some of you did not get this mother in real life. That is all the more reason to be a good mother to yourself. Maybe you need re-mothering.

Your mothering voice is your inner voice. It is the voice of your spirit, your intuition, your inner guide, God, Goddess, Jesus, the Holy Spirit, Mary, Christ Consciousness, soul, mentor, or your best friend. If mother doesn't work for you, choose another word. But let the M of SOFT AIM bring you to your healthiest voice, the one that embodies both wisdom and compassion. This is a voice that will always lead you to a sense of greater well-being.

It might feel strange at first to talk to yourself in this voice. The fact is, you have lots of inner voices: the critic, the rebel, the inner child, the "hell with it voice" etc. We routinely speak to ourselves as if we are at least two people. For example, how often do you hear some-one lament, "I just couldn't get anything accomplished today." Or, "I know what I am supposed to be doing, but I just don't do it." Who is the *you* that is not accomplishing anything today? Who is the *you* that simply does not do what she knows she needs to do?" What is her relationship to you? Often times the other voice is the critic. But part of us, albeit a sometimes small part, knows this is not healthy. Who is the *you* that recognizes your own self-criticism as harmful?

We need to listen to the back and forth dialogue, alternating our awareness between the small voice of our thoughts and stories and the expansive voice of our healthy self. Mothering is about strength-ening the healthy voice. This is the voice we need. This is the voice our spirit longs for. This is the voice of recovery.

Again, I must encourage you to journal your voices in second person. It is easy to think the automatic, uninvestigated voice in our mind is rational and speaking truth. Writing our thoughts down often makes the foolishness of this voice apparent. It also helps our healthy voice decipher the underlying message of the chatter. For example: "Everyone hates me. I am so stupid". Deciphered: Our internal self feels hurt and inadequate and needs encouragement.

One of the benefits of tapping into the voice of wisdom and compassion is that it will lead us to our true self. The longer we have had our disordered relationship with food, the more we need this healthy voice. In our quest for thinness, we become the glutton or the saint. We think we are on a voyage to a better, thinner life where we will *finally* be all that we can be. The fact is, life is happening now.

In my practice, I often counsel women who say they want recovery with all their heart, but then they sabotage their success at every turn. They fear what they say they want. They fear recovery will turn them into selfish, lying cheats. They will change too much. They will have an affair, become a terrible mother, and so on.

Developing your mothering voice is your guide, your wisdom and your intuitive knowing. Developing this voice gives you a stronger moral compass that enables you to live in alignment with your values. It allows you to live congruently. After all, if your belief system says to treat others fairly, but you currently do not apply that to yourself, you are not congruent. Not investigating your thoughts hurts you in other ways too. If you have fears about poverty and find a wallet, even though you have a value of honesty, you may keep the money because you are still a slave to your fears. If you value fairness, but are afraid to intervene when you see something unfair happening, you are out of alignment again. Living in alignment means that you are authentic and living by your principles more, not less. The Mothering voice allows you to become a true expression of who you are.

Diets, are scary. If you have put weight on to keep your marriage safe, you may fear you will wander when you lose the weight. And as is often the case, you scare yourself so much, that you gain the weight back.

If you are to lose the weight, you must develop the healthy self-mothering voice and all of SOFT AIM. This is the way of recovery. Diets, which work only on the physical body, are missing half of the problem: your thinking. Research supports the mind and body connection.[1] Why would losing weight be any different? You need to work on your physical and emotional health simultaneously. The guidelines of recovery and SOFT AIM give you those tools for recovery of body and mind.

Self-Care and Self-Mothering

Why use this voice? This is likely the voice you would use to help a friend who is struggling. You may even use it to help a stranger. Why not extend the same kindness to yourself?

Another benefit of becoming acquainted with our inner mothering voice is that this is the only way to learn to discern real fear from imagined fear. You can't completely banish your fears. They help keep you alive. But wouldn't it be nice to be able to trust yourself to tell and trust the difference between your false fears and real fear.

You must develop your healthy mothering voice because you have spent too much time in your lower brain and in your logical left hemisphere. The left hemisphere is good for many things, but it is also the home of what the Buddhists call "monkey mind." It is full of stories and judgments and opinions. It is good for identifying a problem and a goal but not for solving it. It is often negatively biased and causes more emotional distress. It can't see the forest for the trees. We are not sure exactly what the source of our healthy voice is, but it probably resides on the right side of the higher brain.

Your inner guidance in the form of self-mothering is always available. At first it might be fuzzy but you can develop this voice by practice and by journaling. The Mothering voice is your most valuable tool and it will guide you in the right direction. She has been there all along. You need only to be still and listen.

Ways to Strengthen our Self-Mothering/Intuitive Voice

- Practice Mindfulness. You can do this any way that you like. A formal practice is great, but just pausing throughout the day to become present, taking a few breaths and stilling yourself is also advantageous.

- Develop a creative life. So often when we are in our disordered relationship with food, we neglect other pursuits. Best-selling author Elizabeth Gilbert, in her book, *Big Magic*,[2] suggests we not wait for passion, but just follow our curiosity. Are you drawn to visual arts, music, writing or gardening? One of the ways we recover is through self-care. If food is our only go-to, we stand little hope of letting it go. We need other pursuits, other abandons, and other ways to care for ourselves.
- Listen to your dreams. Since so many of our thoughts and behaviors run on unconscious patterns, our dreams can be full of information.
- Consult your body. Our feelings are messengers that reside in our body. If you make a decision that is making you queasy, your intuitive self may be speaking to you. Listen.
- I am a huge proponent of walking outdoors in nature. We need to unhook from technology to hear our inner guidance.
- Know your values. What values and character traits are important to you? Are you living in accordance with them? Being out of sync with the values you profess is a signal that you are being run by fear and not listening to your inner mothering voice.
- Trust you intuition. Test it out in small ways. Stop making light of it. Listen.

Practice

Close your eyes. Acknowledge that you do have an inner voice. Apologize for being gone for so long. Tell her you are back and ready to listen. Place your awareness where you think your inner voice resides. For many it is the heart area, but there is no right or wrong. (I think my intuition is in my gut.) Ask this voice to talk to you. Be patient; it may take a while. She may be asleep from the boredom of never being asked for help or never being listened to. Follow her guidance for something small. See what happens. Write it down.

Remember, mothering is not about trying to make everything

perfect. That *trying* is just more strife and striving. It is an attempt to control life. You are aiming, but softly. The self-mothering voice will help you override automatic thoughts and discern real fears from imagined ones. Mothering is a presence, a source to tap into for clarity and wisdom. Your true voice is in the stillness, the being. Let it go. Let it all go. Trust the process. Trust your inner mother and relax into recovery. It is a long ride.

Journal Assignment

1. How will I allow my recovery to be a doorway to better understanding myself and healing from past hurts and traumas?
2. How will I allow my recovery to help me grow spiritually as I grow in my intuitive self? How can I become a person who is capable of self-trust and confidence?
3. What fears, if any, do I have about letting the intuitive voice of the mother guide me?
4. Will I trust the path?
5. Am I willing to at least entertain the notion that there is a force greater than my busy mind available to guide me towards my highest good?

CHAPTER 13

Pulling It Together

> You were sick, but now you're well again, and there's work
> to do.
>
> *-Kurt Vonnegut*

Unfortunately, many of us read but don't do. How will you assure
your follow-through? That is much of what this final chapter is about.
In my experience, the difference between the talkers and the doers,
those who are moved to action instead of just reading books is not a
lack of competence, but rather a lack of confidence. You have to believe you have the power to change your life in order to do so.

It is time to take all of the tools you have read about and put them
to use. Hopefully by now you are practicing and having some success
with these techniques: (or skills, or actions)

- Becoming aware of and changing self-defeating inner talk
- Eating when hungry
- Practicing stopping eating when satiated
- Using SOFT AIM to develop emotional resilience

It takes diligence and determination to use these tools. As stated
earlier, most disordered eating behaviors run at an unconscious level.
Making the unconscious conscious is not a small feat. You will also

need a great deal of patience and self-compassion to stay on this path. In this chapter you are going to learn more techniques to handle your emotions as opposed to eating through them. As you have learned, the most difficult time to use these skills will be the moment when you are feeling compulsive.

Let's Review.

1. When you recognize yourself wanting to eat when you are not hungry, STOP! Your lower brain is over-activated and trying to run you. Retreat to a quiet place. Take out your journal.

2. Put on your interested OBSERVER hat. Remember that by observing you are protecting yourself from being hijacked and, therefore, controlled by the emotion. You are simply observing from a neutral stance, no judgment whatsoever.

3. From this place, gently identify what FEELING is behind the compulsive craving. Sit with it non-judgmentally. Find it in your body. Let's say for example, the feeling is sadness; let's assume the feeling is in your heart. For this assignment you gently place your hand on your heart and say, "Hello sadness. What message are you bringing me today?" Just saying "hello" to your emotion in this gentle and interested way; you have separated yourself from its intensity. You are putting your healthy self in charge, for it is your healthy self that has asked this question. Write down the emotion. Keep it short and simple. Emotions are just words like: happy, sad, lonely, anxious, afraid, overwhelmed, etc.

4. Travel up to your brain where your THOUGHT resides. What is the thought or story that creates this emotion? Put it in second person to hear it more clearly. Do not censor the thought. Let it be as judgmental and irrational as it may be.

5. Next, consciously ALLOW your findings. Allowing does not imply agreement. Too often we run from the feeling and the thoughts and are willing to do anything to calm ourselves again. In the situation of compulsive eating, we seek comfort and calm through food. You can't change anything until

you understand the situation and identify the challenges that confront you. A physical way to help yourself let go and allow is to simply clench and unclench your fists as you remind yourself to allow.

6. Once you have accepted where you are, you can INVESTIGATE the thought. Is it balanced or is there a more balanced way to look at things? Your investigation should be without judgment as well. Think fair and balanced.

7. Lastly, you need to compassionately comfort yourself in a loving MOTHER to child way. Remember a good mother is not permissive nor punitive, but is both fair and loving. You must use the voice you would use for your most cherished friend.

Hopefully, the following example will clarify this process even further. Let's say Melissa has been working on recovery for a while and recognizes that although she is feeling compulsive towards food, she is not physically hungry. She finds a quiet place, sits with her journal, and goes through the SOFT AIM process as follows:

STOP: Melissa recognizes she is in trouble. She STOPS and focuses by taking three deep breaths, slowly saying "peace" as she inhales and "calm" on the exhale.

OBSERVE: She is curious and open to understand what is going on.

FEELING: In her observing non-judgmental way, Melissa inquires as to what feeling she is experiencing? She locates anxiety in her throat. It is a tightness, a feeling of constriction.

THOUGHT: Melissa writes down the thoughts that create anxiety in her journal in second person. "This is terrible. They pretty much said there is going to be a lay-off at the plant. You are going to lose everything. You cannot afford this. How will you ever find another job at your age? And you are going to lose your health insurance too! Then you are really screwed." This running commentary could go on for a while. Let it yammer as long as it needs to. Ask, "Is that all or is there more?" Let this voice go until it is done.

ALLOW: Melissa writes her feelings and accompanying thoughts out on paper. Now she can take a breath and accept that this is the feeling and this is the story. As the saying goes, "It is what it is."

INVESTIGATE: Melissa is accessing both her right empathic brain and left logical brain to assist with problem solving and finding the most balanced way to think about the situation. Investigation must be done with the last part of the acronym, "Mother".

MOTHER: Melissa investigates the story with compassion and curiosity. "Sweetheart, let's just take one step at a time. While this may happen, you would get unemployment which would pay most of the bills. You could cut back on a few expenses. You have time to find another job. Let's look at your bills to see what you owe and maybe make a preliminary, just in case, plan. Now, what do you need? What would help this feeling of anxiety tonight?" Melissa realizes that it would be best not to be alone tonight. She calls a few friends and finds someone that can meet her and talk.

It is important that we give ourselves what we need. Recovery needs to look promising, not just like more deprivation. If we are not giving ourselves the numbing of compulsive eating, we need to give ourselves something else. Maybe, as in this case, it is to call a friend, or to cry, or to ask for a hug. Maybe it is the distraction of a movie or good book. When we decide what we need, we must do our best to follow through with action. We need to give to ourselves what we would give to a friend.

Journal Assignment
1. Can you be brave, optimistic, and willing to do whatever it takes to recover? This is not for the faint of heart.
2. What within you is holding you back from recovery?
3. Do you feel worthy of recovery?

4. What do you gain from staying in your dysfunctional relationship with food and your body?

5. Are you willing to give up numbing comfort for what you can gain in recovery?

6. Write your own recovery plan. What tools will you use? Who will be your support?

More Coping Skills

Because I think we need an arsenal of coping skills, I offer the following to use in addition to SOFT AIM:

- EFT-The Emotional Freedom Technique, or EFT, developed by Gary Craig in the early 1990's is a widely used psychological acupressure technique.[1] It is useful for reducing the moment of cravings, reducing or eliminating pain, or letting go of difficult emotional states. It calms the amygdala, thereby reducing anxiety. It is very easy to learn. I would suggest reading more about EFT and possibly buying one of the books listed in the recommended reading section to learn more. You can even download apps to teach you how to use it.

- *The Work* by Byron Katie[2] is a very effective tool for changing beliefs and learning the art of allowing. You can even download worksheets on TheWork.com

- EMDR-Eye Movement Desensitization and Reprocessing.[3] This is a therapeutic technique that should only be done by a trained professional. It is specifically used to treat unresolved trauma. Clients recall a distressing image while receiving specific sensory input.

- Breathing techniques. A variety of techniques have been discussed throughout this book. Find one or two that work for you.

- Mindfulness. Practice presence. Be aware of the sights and sounds around you. Notice the water on your hands when you wash dishes, the feel of your legs on the chair, the life in your right hand. Anything that brings you into the now is mindfulness. You might consider joining a meditation group.

- Prayer. Learning to pray for willingness is especially useful in recovery. As the slogan in the 12 step movement goes, "It was your own bad thinking that got you here." The mothering part of SOFT AIM is our way of turning it over, letting it go and surrendering to a higher wisdom.
- Complementary medicine modalities. Get massages regularly. Energy healing, using herbs, Reiki, or essential oils can all be useful in calming the mind.
- Exercise. It has been proven that exercise lowers stress. Many compulsive eaters have tendencies to over exercise once they start. Always give your body at least one day off, and do not exercise over 1-1½ hours.
- Walks outdoors. I love walking outdoors. Getting away from technology and immersing ourselves in nature naturally lowers our stress.
- Journaling. As we discussed earlier in the book, putting our feelings in writing is another way to figure out solutions to issues and calm ourselves.
- Distraction. Sometimes all we need is a break. This could be a nap, a funny movie or lunch with a friend, to name but a few.

Find what works for you and remember SOFT AIM.

Trusting the Process

Life is a journey. If you picked up this book your recovery is likely part of that journey. I like walking the labyrinth because it reminds me of the journey we are all on and how similar recovery is to a labyrinth path. Recovery can feel meandering, taking us in circles and alternately in spirals and sharp turns. If we understand that we are on a sacred journey, we can trust that the path is purposeful. Like the labyrinth, we can't see the outcome or destination that the path is taking us. Still we move forward. Although we do not know what is ahead, we trust the process. And like the process of SOFT AIM, we are not trying to control or force anything. We intend. That is aiming softly. Remember, fear contracts intention. Like a walk in a labyrinth, we are simply putting the next step forward.

My wish for you is that SOFT AIM will provide you with an important tool to face the challenges of disordered eating. If you are prepared to *stop* and *observe* your *feelings* and *thoughts* and to *allow, investigate,* and listen to your healthy self-*mothering* voice, you, dear reader, are on the road to recovery.

Recommended Reading

Books Specific to Recovery

1. *Eating in the Light of the Moon*, How Women Can Transform Their Relationship with Food Through Myths, Metaphors, and Storytelling by *Anita Johnston (Gurze Books, 1ˢᵗ edition 2000)*
2. *Feeding the Hungry Heart: The Experience of Compulsive Eating* by Geneen Roth (Plume reissue edition 1993)
3. *Goodbye Ed, Hello Me*, by *Jenni Schaefer* (McGraw-Hill Education; 1 edition July 19, 2009)
4. *It's Not About Food: End Your Obsession with Food and Weight*, by *Carol Normandi and Lauralee Roark* (Tarcher Perigee; Revised, Expanded ed. edition December 2, 2008)
5. *Overcoming Overeating* by Jane Hirshmann <u>Carol H. Munter</u> (OO Publishing 2010)
6. *The Food and Feelings Workbook, A Full Course Meal on Emotional Health* by Karen R, Koenig (Gurze Books; 1st edition January 15, 2007)
7. *The Rules of Normal Eating,* by Karen Koenig (Gurze Books; 1 edition January 14, 2005)
8. *When Food Is Love,* by Geneen Roth (Plume; Reissue edition July 1, 1992)

Books to Nourish the Soul

1. *Awakening Joy: 10 Steps that will Put You on the Road to Real Happiness* by James Baraz and Shoshana Alexander (Parallax Press November 15, 2012)
2. *Big Magic* by Elizabeth Gilbert (Riverhead Books 2015)
3. *Bouncing Back: Rewiring Your Brain for Maximum Resilience and Well-Being* by Linda Graham New World Library; 4.9.2013 edition (April 9, 2013)
4. *Broken Open How Difficult Times Can Help Us Grow* by Elizabeth Lesser (Villard; Reprint edition June 14, 2005)
5. *Daring Greatly: How the Courage to Be Vulnerable Transforms the Way We Live, Love, Parent, and Lead* by Brene Brown (Avery; 1st edition September 11, 2012)
6. *Emotional Intelligence*-Daniel Goleman (Bantam 2012)
7. *Finding your own North Star: Claiming the Life you were meant to Live* by Martha Beck (Harmony; Reprint edition January 29, 2002)
8. *Highly Sensitive People: Guide to survive overwhelming relationships* by Heidi Sawyer (The Heidi Sawyer Group November 19, 2013)
9. *Loving What Is: Four Questions That Can Change Your Life* by Byron Katie and Stephen Mitchell. (Harmony 2002)
10. *Peace Is Every Step: The Path of Mindfulness in Everyday Life* by Thich Nhat Hanh (Bantam March 1, 1992)
11. *Radical Acceptance: Embracing Your Life with the Heart of a Buddha* by Tara Brach. (Bantam 2004)
12. *Rising Strong How the Ability to Reset Transforms the Way We Live, Love, Parent, and Lead* by Brene Brown Spiegel & Grau; Reprint edition (August 25, 2015)
13. *What's in the Way Is The Way: A Practical Guide to Waking up to Life* by Mary O'Malley (Sounds True January 1, 2016)
14. *The Tapping Solution for Weight Loss & Body Confidence: A Woman's Guide to Stressing Less, Weighing Less, and Loving

More by Jessica Ortner (Hay House, Inc.; Reprint edition (October 27, 2015)

15. *The Tapping Solution. A Revolutionary Program for Stress Free Living* by Nick Ortner (Hay House, Inc.; 8th ed. edition September 16, 2014)

16. *The Road Less Traveled A New Psychology of Love, Traditional Values and Spiritual Growth* by M. Scott Peck (Touchstone; Anniversary edition February 4, 2003)

17. *The Fear Cure Cultivating Courage as Medicine for the Body, Mind, and Soul* by Lissa Rankin, M.D. (Hay House February 24, 2015)

Notes

Chapter 1
Welcome to the Wild Ride

1. Christelle Audeta T. and Robin D. Everall, *Therapist self-disclosure and the therapeutic relationship: a phenomenological study from the client perspective* (Faculty of Education, University of Ottawa)

2. J.W. Pennebaker, *Writing about emotional experiences as a therapeutic process* (Psychological Science, Vol. 8, No. 3 (May, 1997), pp. 162-166

Chapter 2
Waking Up

1. Dan Siegal, *The Developing Mind, How Relationships and the Brain Interact to Shape Who We Are* (The Guilford Press, 2nd edition)

2. Louis Cozolino, *The Neuroscience of Human Relationships: Attachment and the Developing Social Brain* (Norton Series on Interpersonal Neurobiology, 2nd edition)

3. Paul Rozin, Edward B. Royzman, *Negativity Bias, Negativity Dominance, and Contagion* by (Department of Psychology and Solomon Asch Center for Study of Ethnopolitical Conflict University of Pennsylvania)

4. Joseph LeDoux, *Synaptic Self: How Our Brains Become Who We Are.* Penguin Books (January 28, 2003)

5. Jenni Schaefer, *Goodbye ED, Hello Me: Recover from Your Eating Disorder and Fall in Love with Life* (McGraw-Hill Education; 1 edition July 19, 2009)
6. Jean Kilbourne, *Killing us Softly: Advertising and It's Effect on Women* 1999. (DVD)

Chapter 3
Letting your Hunger Guide you

1. Geneen Roth, *Breaking Free from Compulsive Eating* (Plume 1993)

Chapter 4
Enough Already

1. Ancel Keyes, *The Minnesota Semi-Starvation Study* (Minneapolis: University of Minnesota 1950)
2. K. Spiegel, E. Tasali E, P. Penev P, E.Cauter, *Sleep curtailment in healthy young men is associated with decreased leptin levels, elevated ghrelin levels, and increased hunger and appetite* (University of Chicago, Chicago, Illinois, USA 2004)

Chapter 5
SOFT AIM

1. P.M. Peeke, G.P. Chrousos, *Hypercortisolism and Obesity* (Ann NY Academy Science 1995)
2. Sara W. Lazar, Catherine E. Kerr, Rachel H. Wasserman, Jeremy R. Gray, Douglas N. Greve, Michael T. Treadway, Metta McGarvey, Brian T. Quinn, Jeffery A. Dusek, Herbert Benson, Scott L. Rauch, Christopher I. Moore, and Bruce Fischl, *Meditation experience is associated with increased cortical thickness* (Neuroreport 2005)
3. Daniel M. Wegner, *Ironic Processes of Mental Control* (Psychological Review,1994)
4. Viktor Frankl, *Man's Search for Meaning:An Introduction to Logotherapy* (Beacon Press; 1st edition June 1, 2006)

5. Kristin Neff, *Self-Compassion: The Proven Power of being Kind to Yourself* (Harper Collins, 2011)

6. Tosha Silver, *Outrageous Openness: Letting the Divine Take the Lead* (Atria Books; April 21, 2014)

Chapter 6
S is for Stop

1. Bruce Lipton, Ph.D, *The Biology of Belief: Unleashing the Power of Consciousness, Matter & Miracles* (Hay House 2015)

Chapter 7
Observe, aka "Isn't that Interesting?"

1. James Baraz and Shoshana Alexander, *Awakening Joy: 10 Steps that will Put You on the Road to Real Happiness* (Bantam Books New York)

Chapter 8
F is for Feeling

1. Jane Hirschmann and Carol H. Munter, *Overcoming Overeating* (OO Publishing 2010)

2. I.K. Broverman, D. M. Broverman, F.E. Clarkson, P.S. Rosenkrantz, & S.R. Vogel, *Sex-role stereotypes and clinical judgments of mental health* (Journal of Consulting and Clinical Psychology, 1970)

3. Daniel Goleman, *Emotional Intelligence* (Bantam 2012)

Chapter 9
T is for Thoughts

1. Robert Burton, M.D. *A Skeptic's Guide to the Mind: What Neuroscience Can and Cannot Tell Us About Ourselves* (St. Martin's Press 2013)

2. Belinda S Lennerz, David C Alsop, Laura M Holsen, Emily Stern, Rafael Rojas, Cara B Ebbeling, Jill M Goldstein, and David S Ludwig. *Effects of dietary glycemic index on brain*

regions related to reward and craving in men (Am Journal of Clinical Nutr, June 26, 2013)

3. Jill Bolte Taylor, *My Stroke of Insight: A Brain Scientist's Personal Journey* Ph.D.(Penguin Books 2008)

Chapter 10
A is for Allow

1. Byron Katie and Stephen Mitchell, *Loving What Is: Four Questions That Can Change Your Life* . (Harmony 2002)
2. Mary O'Malley, *What's in the way is the way* (Sounds True 2016)
3. Kelly Koerner and Marsha Linehan. *Doing Dialectical Behavioral Therapy: A Practical Guide* (Guilford Press 2012)
4. Tara Brach *Radical Acceptance: Embracing Your Life With the Heart of a Buddha* (Bantam 2004)

Chapter 11
Investigate Like CSI

1. Byron Katie, Stephen Mitchell, *Loving What Is: Four Questions That Can Change Your Life* (Harmony 2002)

Chapter 12
M is for Mother

1. Science Daily, *Mechanism between Mind-Body Connection Discovered* July 16, 2008 University of California
2. Elizabeth Gilbert *Big Magic: Creative Living Beyond Fear* (Riverhead Books 2015)

Chapter 13
Pulling It Together

1. Gary Craig *EFT Handbook* (Energy Psychology Press; 2nd edition (March 15, 2011)
2. Byron Katie and Stephen Mitchell, *Loving What Is: Four Questions That Can Change Your Life*. (Harmony 2002)

3. <u>Francine Shapiro</u>, <u>Margot Silk Forrest</u>, *EMDR: The Breakthrough Therapy for Overcoming Anxiety, Stress, and Trauma* by (Basic Books; Updated edition September 13, 2016)

CPSIA information can be obtained
at www.ICGtesting.com
Printed in the USA
FFOW02n1815220617
37038FF